Obsessive–Compulsive Disorder

Psychological and Pharmacological Treatment

T0332975

Obsessive–Compulsive Disorder

Psychological and
Pharmacological Treatment

EDITED BY

MATIG MAVISSAKALIAN
SAMUEL M. TURNER
AND
LARRY MICHELSON

Western Psychiatric Institute and Clinic
University of Pittsburgh School of Medicine
Pittsburgh, Pennsylvania

Plenum Press • New York and London

Library of Congress Cataloging in Publication Data

Main entry under title:

Obessive-compulsive disorder.

Includes bibliographies and index.
1. Obessive-compulsive neurosis—Treatment. 2. Psychotherapy. 3. Obsessive-compulsive neurosis—Chemotherapy. I. Mavissakalian, Matig, 1943–   . II. Turner, Samuel M., 1944–   . III. Michelson, Larry, 1952–   . [DNLM: 1. Obsessive-Compulsive Disorders—therapy. WM 176 0145]
RC533.O27   1985   616.85′227   84-26395
ISBN 0-306-41850-9

©1985 Plenum Press, New York
A Division of Plenum Publishing Corporation
233 Spring Street, New York, N.Y. 10013

Contributors

JAMBUR ANANTH, Director, Psychopharmacology Harbor, UCLA Medical Center, University of California at Los Angeles, Torrance, CA

E. B. FOA, Temple University, Department of Psychiatry, EPPI, 3300 Henry Avenue, Philadelphia, PA

MATIG MAVISSAKALIAN, Western Psychiatric Institute and Clinic, University of Pittsburgh School of Medicine, 3811 O'Hara Street, Pittsburgh, PA

LARRY MICHELSON, Western Psychiatric Institute and Clinic, University of Pittsburgh School of Medicine, 3811 O'Hara Street, Pittsburgh, PA

B. J. OZAROW, Department of Psychology, Aquinas College, Grand Rapids, MI

S. JACK RACHMAN, Department of Psychology, University of British Columbia, Vancouver, British Columbia, Canada

LEON SALZMAN, Georgetown University Medical School, 1800 R Street, NW, Washington, DC

PETER E. SIFNEOS, Department of Psychiatry, Harvard Medical
School, and Beth Israel Hospital, Boston, MA

G. S. STEKETEE, Temple University, Department of Psychiatry,
EPPI, 3300 Henry Avenue, Philadelphia, PA

SAMUEL TURNER, Western Psychiatric Institute and Clinic,
University of Pittsburgh School of Medicine, 3811 O'Hara
Street, Pittsburgh, PA

Preface

Recent advances in behavioral and biological treatments have raised the hopes and expectations of patients and clinicians alike in regard to obsessive-compulsive disorder—one of the most disabling, crippling, and resistant conditions in psychiatry. In addition to their therapeutic efficacy, these new treatments have also opened new conceptual perspectives, thus complementing the traditional psychological theories of obsessive-compulsive disorder. Therefore, it is timely for these various conceptual frameworks and the treatment modalities they engender to be integrated and synthesized in the present volume. To this end, eminent scholars in their respective areas were invited to contribute to this book, which we hope will symbolize and—in some measure—actualize the spirit of collaboration required if we are to fully comprehend the complex nature of this disorder as well as to address existing therapeutic challenges.

In Chapter 1, Rachman sets the stage by providing an overview of the conceptual and therapeutic issues of obsessive-compulsive disorder. This is followed by an in-depth review of the behavioral interventions from which Foa

vii

and colleagues successfully distill the specific therapeutic processes of exposure and response prevention. In the third chapter, Sifneos deals with the psychodynamic factors underlying obsessive-compulsive phenomena and details his innovative technique of brief, anxiety-provoking psychotherapy aimed specifically at the obsessional state. In the next chapter, Salzman, commenting on the psychological treatments of obsessive-compulsive disorder, emphasizes the necessity for effective symptom removal as well as the elucidation of the meaning that symptoms and their eventual relinquishment have for the patient. In the fifth chapter, Ananth reviews the pharmacological and psychosurgical interventions that pave the way for the biological investigations of obsessive-compulsive disorder. In the final chapter, we identify and discuss controversial aspects of the phenomenology, classification, and treatment of this disorder that ostensibly require further study.

Though the scholarly reviews of the literature should make this book relevant reading to any student of obsessive-compulsive disorder, the volume ought to have special appeal to psychiatrists and clinical psychologists in training. In reading these pages, we urge the reader to put aside orientational preferences and to approach each model as having something specific to offer. No one model is perfect, and no single treatment is completely effective. There is reason for optimism, although it must be tempered with the knowledge that our understanding of etiology still lags far behind advances made in the treatment of obsessive-compulsive phenomena.

We wish to thank the administration of Western Psychiatric Institute and Clinic in Pittsburgh as this book is based, in part, on a symposium held there. We would also like to express our gratitude to the senior editor at Plenum, Eliot Werner, for his support during the project. Finally, we dedicate this book to clinicians everywhere who, with open minds, recognize and apply the specific merits of behavioral, pharmacological, and dynamic therapies to the betterment of their obsessive-compulsive patients.

MATIG MAVISSAKALIAN
SAMUEL M. TURNER
LARRY MICHELSON

Contents

CHAPTER 2

Behavior Therapy with Obsessive-Compulsives: From
Theory to Treatment 49

E. B. Foa, G. S. Steketee, and B. J. Ozarow

CHAPTER 3

Short-Term Dynamic Psychotherapy for Patients
Suffering from an Obsessive-Compulsive Disorder ... 131

Peter E. Sifneos

Chapter 4

Comments on the Psychological Treatment of
Obsessive-Compulsive Patients 155

Leon Salzman

CHAPTER 5

CHAPTER 6

1

An Overview of Clinical and Research Issues in Obsessional-Compulsive Disorders

S. JACK RACHMAN

CHARACTERISTICS OF OBSESSIONS AND COMPULSIONS

Since the introduction of the concept of obsessional-compulsive disorder (OCD) well over a hundred years ago, the definition of the disorder has produced little controversy. The main features are difficult to mistake, and recent research has enabled us to clarify and review the concept. Jaspers's (1963) definition is representative and comprehensive.

> In a strict sense of the term, compulsive thoughts, impulses, etc., should be confined to anxieties or impulses which can be experienced by the individual as an incessant preoccupation, though he is convinced of the *groundlessness* of the anxiety, the *senselessness* of the impulse and the *impossibility* of the notion. Thus, the compulsive events, strictly speaking, are all such

---

S. JACK RACHMAN • Department of Psychology, University of British Columbia, Vancouver, British Columbia, Canada V6T 1Y7

1

events the existence of which is strongly resisted by the individual in the first place, and the *content* of which appears to him as groundless, meaningless or relatively incomprehensible.(p. 134, original emphasis).

Few substantial changes have been introduced into that definition, but we are now in a position to specify the relevant phenomena more closely and to say more about the content of the disorders and the relations between different aspects of the problems experienced by the affected person.

An *obsession* is an intrusive, repetitive thought, image, or impulse that is unacceptable or unwanted and gives rise to subjective resistance. It generally produces distress and is characteristically difficult to remove or control. The affected person generally acknowledges the senselessness of the impulse or idea. The content of an obsession is repugnant, worrying, blasphemous, obscene, nonsensical, or all of these. The person might be repetitively troubled by the thought that he or she might have killed someone, or by images of mutilated babies, or by doubts about whether he or she is moral or intensely evil, about whether he or she might have a compulsive urge to expose his or her genitals in public, or shout obscenities, and so forth. In an analysis of 81 OCD patients, Akhtar, Wig, Verma, Pershod, and Verma (1975) found that the content of obsessional material could be broken down into five categories, which are given here in descending order of frequency: dirt and contamination, aggression, orderliness of inanimate objects, sex, and religion. In support of Lewis's (1966) claim that the content of the obsession is of little use prognostically, they found no relation between content and outcome.

Compulsions are repetitive, stereotyped acts. They may be wholly unacceptable, or more often partly acceptable, but they are regarded by the person as being excessive or exaggerated. They are preceded or accompanied by a subjective sense of compulsion, and they generally provoke subjective resistance. They usually produce distress, and the person can acknowledge the senselessness of his or her activities, when judged in calmer moments. Although the activities are within the person's voluntary control, the urge to carry out the acts can be extremely powerful, and hence the person experiences a sense of diminished volition. The two most common types of compulsive activity, often referred to as *compulsive rituals*, are repetitive cleaning and checking. The classical example of the former type is a person who compulsively checks the security of appliances and of entrances to his or her home.

There is a close and probably causal relationship between compulsive urges and compulsive acts, with the former producing the latter. Obsessions and compulsions are closely related, and in the study by Akhtar and his colleagues, referred to earlier, it was found that 25% of the patients reported having obsessions that were not associated with overt acts. In the study of 150 OCD inpatients, Wilner, Reich, Robins, Fishman, and van Doren (1976) reported that 69% of the patients complained of both obsessions and compulsions, 25% had obsessions only, and a mere 6% had compulsions only.

One can describe a person as having an OCD: (a) if his or her major complaint is the repeated occurrence of an obsession and/or compulsion; (b) if there are accompanying behavioral signs of such experiences; and (c) if the symptoms are associated with distress and impairment of psychological functioning (socially, occupationally, sexually, etc.). The experience of subjective compulsion, the report of internal resistance, and the presence of insight are generally regarded as the three indicators of an obsessional-compulsive disorder. Aside from their obsessional-compulsive symptoms, the affected person generally has what is described somewhat clumsily as an "intact personality." These working definitions of the major phenomena encountered in these disorders are not without their difficulties (cf. Rachman & Hodgson, 1980), but they will suffice for present purposes.

OCD can be both distressing and disabling, sometimes to the point of destroying a person's life. Clinical examples of severe disorders are given by Meyer (1966), Jaspers (1963), and by Rachman and Hodgson (1980), among others. Although the problems that characterize these disorders are probably widespread in the general population, they only become matters of clinical concern when the intensity and/or frequency of the problem becomes a matter of distress or disablement. In conventional terms, OCD has a relatively low incidence, as is discussed in the next section.

Briefly, the necessary and sufficient conditions for describing repetitive behavior as *compulsive* are an experienced sense of pressure to act and attributing this pressure to internal sources. The occurrence of resistance is a confirmatory feature but is neither necessary nor sufficient. The necessary and sufficient features for defining a repetitive thought, impulse, or image as *obsessional* are intrusiveness, internal attribution, unwantedness, and difficulty of control. The confirmatory indicators are resistance and an alien quality. An obsessional-compulsive disorder is one in which the person's major complaint is of distress caused by obsessions or compulsions. The overt indicators are repetitive, stereotyped behaviors and a degree of psychological and social impairment associated with the complaints.

In conventional diagnostic practice, one of the most difficult distinctions to draw is that between an obsession and an overvalued idea (e.g., "Are the dark patches on my skin early signs of cancer?" 'My bowels are obstructed/distorted"). In view of Foa's observations on failures in treatment (see Chapter 2), the distinction can be of predictive significance. The only other point on which disagreements arise with any frequency is whether or not the person's report of internal resistance to the obsessions or compulsions is a necessary feature of the disorder. The findings of Rachman and Hodgson (1980) and Stern and Cobb (1978) suggest that resistance is a common and significant indicator but not a necessary one.

The study of these disorders is of considerable interest because in many ways they are the purest examples of abnormal behaviors. People whose behavior is in most respects well within rational borders repetitively carry out acts that they recognize to be senseless—to a considerable extent they are executing urges against their rational inclinations. For many patients, the relatively uncontrolled repetitive conduct of essentially irrational acts is the greatest source of distress. These disorders are relatively uncommon but can be extraordinarily distressing for the affected person and often for large numbers of friends and relatives who can rarely escape the adverse consequences of this distressing and disabling behavior.

COURSE OF DISORDER

A number of admirably comprehensive reviews of the disorder have been carried out, and there is a large measure of agreement between the accounts given by different authors (Black, 1974; Goodwin, Guze, & Robins, 1969; Kringlen, 1970; Lewis, 1936, 1966; Rachman & Hodgson, 1980; Salzman & Thaler, 1981; Templer, 1972; Wilner et al., 1976). In summary form, the conclusions drawn by these reviewers include the following. Obsessional-compulsive disorders usually begin in late adolescence or early adulthood; in one- to two- thirds of the reported cases, significant life events are associated with the onset of the problem; a majority of patients report having had a variety of neurotic problems during childhood; people with fully developed OCD usually are socially isolated; and although the general prognosis is, in conventional terms, rather unfavorable, the suicide rate for these patients is lower than it is for patients with other psychiatric difficulties. There is an intimate relationship between depression and OCD.

Demographic data are provided by Hare, Price, and Slater (1972) and by Black (1974). The percentage of psychiatric outpatients diagnosed as OCD lies between 0.3% and 0.6%, but they provide a slightly higher percentage of inpatient admissions than do patients with other forms of neurotic disorder. It is a rather more serious disorder than the general run of neurotic problems. Although males and females are equally represented in the demographic data, it seems probable from information collected by Rachman and Hodgson that males and females tend to develop slightly different forms of the disorder. People with these disorders also tend to be socially isolated and have a high celibacy rate, particularly the males. Both males and females tend to marry at an older age than other types of psychiatric patients, and they have a low fertility rate. In a series of 83 patients, we found an interesting associaton between cleaning compulsions and gender (Rachman & Hodgson, 1980). No less than 86% of the compulsive cleaners were female; the ratio of females to males was 6:1. Virtually the only point on which the different reviewers fail to agree is on the "natural" course taken by the disorder. (The natural history or course of a disorder, entirely uninfluenced by therapeutic interventions, is difficult to study, and few patients remain untreated for any length of time.) In Kringlen's (1965) estimation, the spontaneous remission rate is in the region of 25%, but Lo (1967) quotes a figure of 71% for his sample. Discussions of the so-called natural history of the disorder are given by Rachman and Hodgson (1980) and by Rachman and Wilson (1980) who considered the matter in the context of a range of neurotic disorders (see later discussion). They estimated that the spontaneous remission rate for OCD is probably somewhat lower than it is for anxiety states and other neurotic complaints. In these cases, a crude spontaneous remission rate of 65% *within 2 years of onset* is used (cf. Eysenck & Rachman, 1965).

RELATION TO OTHER DISORDERS

For some time, particularly at the turn of the century, it was believed that there was a close association between obsessions and schizophrenia, but the contemporary view, based on fuller and more reliable information, runs contrary to this idea. With minor exceptions, recent evidence is consistent in showing that only a tiny percentage of OCD patients subsequently develop schizophrenia or any other form of psychosis. Moreover, this percentage is no higher than it is for other neurotic disorders (cf. Black, 1974; Kringlen, 1970; Lo, 1967; Pollitt, 1957). Another view that has received little support during the past few years is that of a functional connection between OCD and organic impairment. Those very few cases in which such a connection has been demonstrated, appear to have features that distinguish them from the disorders manifested by people in whom there is no suggestion of an organic dysfunction. The features suggestive of an organic dysfunction include (a) a history of injury, illness, or birth complication; (b) the obsession or compulsion lacks intellectual content; (c) absence of an intentional component; (d) the affected person usually has associated deficits, especially of a cognitive type; and (e) the compulsions have a stereotyped and mechanical quality.

The distinctive features of OCD in relation to other psychiatric disorders include the following. Obsessions are intrusive unwanted thoughts that cause distress and usually provoke internal resistance. Unlike delusions, they are recognized by the affected person to be of internal origin and usually are recognized as being senseless and ego alien. Compulsions are repetitive stereotyped forms of behavior that are preceded or accompanied by a sense of compulsion that is recognized to be of internal origin. Compulsions also are likely to provoke internal resistance and generally are recognized to be senseless. The intrusive ideas or experiences characteristic of *schizophrenia* differ in that they tend to be attributed to external forces, are not regarded by the affected person as being senseless, and seldom provoke the internal resistance characteristic of OCD. The ideas are not necessarily ego alien. The stereotyped behavior associated with *organic dysfunction* may include repetitive ideas or acts, but these acts lack intellectual content or intentionality and have a far more mechanical and primitive quality than the stereotyped activities characteristic of OCD. Obsessions differ from morbid *preoccupations* in that the latter are intrusive and repetitive ideas that tend to be ego syntonic, to be rational but exaggerated, and to be realistic and current. Moreover, they seldom are resisted. The relation between obsessions, compulsions, and *depression* is widely recognized to be of considerable importance (Lewis, 1966; Videbech, 1975; Wilner *et al.*, 1976), but the nature of this association is not clear. Obsessions and depressions can rise independently, and even in instances in which they are associated at the time of onset, they can then develop independent courses. Notwithstanding the often-reported association between obsessions and depression, it should be remembered that there are many cases in which the OCD is neither accompanied by nor preceded by any clear indications of depression (Wilner *et al.*, 1976). Kringlen (1970), in a careful study of 91 patients, found that roughly one-fifth displayed depressive symptoms, whereas in the series reported by Rachman and Hodgson (1980), 55% of the 83 patients were seemingly free of depressive complaints at the onset of the disorder. There were, however, many instances in which an apparent sequence of obsessions leading to depression was encountered. Wilner and his associates (1976) found that the transition from obsessions to depression occurred three times as often (38% of the cases) as did the reverse sequence (11%). It is potentially of practical importance that in the latter group, where the depression preceded the obsession, there was a better prognosis. Notwithstanding the crucial importance of the association between depression and OCD, one should not lose sight of the examples in which this association is not observed. It has already been mentioned that depression is absent in a proportion of obsessional-compulsive disorders, and we also have evidence that in a small minority of cases the disorder is relieved by the onset of depression (Gittelson, 1966). Furthermore, obsessional-compulsive features and depressions can be encountered in association with other types of psychiatric disorders; the association between depression and obsessional-compulsive disorders is not an exclusive one. Some of the theoretical implications of this complex interaction between mood disturbance and disorders of an obsessional-compulsive kind are considered by Rachman and Hodgson (1980, Chapters 8 and 24).

Some recent research on drug treatments of these disorders supports the idea that in many instances the obsessional-compulsive symptoms are maintained by depression, for there is an improvement in the OCD secondary to the relief of depression (Rachman, Cobb, MacDonald, Mawson, Sartory, & Stern, 1979). This finding was not confirmed in the drug study by Thoren, Asberg, Cronholm, Jornestadt, and Traskman (1980), perhaps because the question was not addressed directly. None of their patients had primary depression, the mean depression scores may have been low (the scale used is not widely known or validated), and the putative causal connection remains to be tested directly.

Attention should also be drawn to the close connection between obsessional-compulsive problems and *excessive fear*. Although the relationship between phobias and cleaning compulsions is particularly close, that between phobias and primary obsessional slowness is slender. As far as the common features are concerned, we now have evidence that the psychophysiological responses of many patients to the presentation of phobic and obsessional-compulsive stimuli appear to be similar. In both instances, an increase in autonomic responsiveness is generally observed. Such responsivity is observed to diminish after successful treatment. The subjective responses to phobic and to obsessional-compulsive material involve a similar increment in subjective discomfort. These subjective responses, like the psychophysiological reactions, tend to be diminished after successful treatment. Both phobic and obsessional-compulsive reactions often are associated with extensive avoidance behavior, which is itself diminished after successful treatment. We also have general clinical evidence of excessive fear among OCD patients (Kringlen, 1965; Skoog, 1959; Videbech, 1975). Adult OCD patients give retrospective reports of having experienced excessive fear during childhood. Furthermore, there is an elevated incidence of anxiety neuroses among relatives of OCD patients.

GENESIS

Unfortunately, we have to rely on approximate and unsystematic information in trying to determine the factors that promote and precipitate OCD. For obvious reasons, direct experimental investigations of the genesis of these disorders is confined to animals, but the prominence of the cognitive element in OCD disorders limits the extent to which one can draw generalizations from the findings on animals. Because we are so often obliged to rely on retrospective information, which is typically incomplete, perhaps unreliable, even the foremost question of the mode of onset has not yet been settled. It has been estimated that in many cases no specific point of onset can be determined (Black, 1974; Goodwin *et al.*, 1969). Even in those cases with apparently acute onset, the earlier occurrence of other and possibly related psychological difficulties cannot be excluded. In the Rachman-Hodgson (1980) series of 83 patients, 51% reported an apparently acute onset. There was, however, no significant relationship between mode of onset and therapeutic outcome, nor was there a relationship with the degree of preparedness. On the other hand, the mode of onset was found to be related to the severity of the disorder. Patients whose disorder was rated as less severe were more likely to have experienced a gradual onset. We also encountered a clear distinction between the mode of onset reported by compulsive checkers and compulsive cleaners. Bearing in mind that many of our 83 patients had some elements of both checking and cleaning problems, we learned that 24 out of our 32 compulsive cleaners described a sudden onset of their difficulties. By contrast, 21 of the 29 compulsive checkers said that the onset of their problem was gradual. A useful summary of the conditions that may precipitate OCD is given by Kringlen (1970). For women, among whom the acute onset was more common, typical stresses were pregnancy, abortion, birth of the first child, and family conflicts.

As far as social and genetic transmission of OCD are concerned, it seems improbable that specific patterns of such behavior are transmitted by observational learning or by direct instruction. There remains, however, a strong possibility that these social learning processes play an important part in generating and maintaining general behavior tendencies, such as timidity, overdependence and so on, and that these dispositions provide fertile soil for the growth of obsessions and compulsions. In addition to these social learning influences and the specific precipitants referred to previously, the role of depression has been mentioned. The fourth possible determinant of obsessions and compulsions is that of genetic transmission. The genetic evidence and arguments were admirably presented in excellent texts by Shields (1973), Slater and Cowie (1971), and by Rosenthal (1970). The genetic evidence is mainly of three types: (a) studies of familial incidence; (b) comparison between twins; and (c) studies of adoptive parents and their children. Slater and Cowie (1971) and Rosenthal (1970) concluded that there is evidence indicating an increased frequency of psychiatric disorder among the close relatives of OCD patients but that no specific associations can be detected. For example, Rosenberg (1967) found in a study of 547 first-degree relatives of 144 patients with obsessional neurosis that only 2 relatives could be diagnosed as having a classical obsessional neurosis. There was, however, an elevated incidence of phobic and anxiety states. The evidence from twin research, mainly that by Tienari (1963) and by Inouye (1965), was the subject of understandable criticism and skepticism. Recently, however, there has been a reemphasis in the direction of an important genetic contribution to OCD. The final outcome of this research will be awaited with great interest. Carey (1978), for example, has shown a higher concordance rate among the co-twins of monozygotic twins with obsessional neurosis than among a comparison group of dizygotic twins. In a psychometric study, Murray, Clifford, Fulker, and Smith (1981) reported a considerable genetic contribution to so-called "obsessionality" among 404 pairs of normal twins. They obtained heritability estimates of 0.44 and 0.47 for obsessional traits and symptoms as measured by the Leyton Obsessional Inventory. These estimates are markedly high, but, among other difficulties, it should not be presumed that the scale is a satisfactory measure of traits or symptoms (see the discussion by Rachman & Hodgson, 1980). It remains the case, however, that the elevated incidence of psychiatric disorder among patients with OCD is reasonably well established. It seems, therefore, that the best course to adopt at the present is to concede that there might well be a nonspecific genetic contribution (perhaps in the form of elevated tendencies to develop general neurotic difficulties) and that specific precipitating events, depression, and social transmission can all play a part in promoting OCD. It will be evident from this brief discussion that the genesis of OCD is poorly understood and there is a serious shortage of pertinent and reliable evidence. Unqualified assertions about the causes of OCD should be treated with caution.

TYPES

A broad division can be drawn between the two *main types of compulsive behavior*. Although it is true that many, perhaps most, of the people who manifest OCD will have elements of both of these forms of compulsions, a distinction between checking compulsions and cleaning compulsions can be drawn and justified. Checking and cleaning compulsions share the common features of an internal sense of pressure, repetitive and stereotyped actions, a commonly experienced feeling of resistance, and partial irrationality, and they are both inclined to produce distress or embarrassment. Checking compulsions usually are oriented to the future and often are intended to prevent harm from coming to someone. For the most part, they can be construed as a form of (preventive) active avoidance behavior. Cleaning compulsions have, in addition, a significant element of passive avoidance behavior, which, when it fails, tends to generate escape behavior. The immediate purpose of carrying out a cleaning ritual is restorative, and it may also have a longer term preventive aim. Cleaning compulsions share some important similarities with phobias. Checking rituals more often than cleaning rituals are associated with doubting and indecisiveness, take a long time to complete, have a slow onset, evoke internal resistance, and are likely to be accompanied by feelings of anger or tension. There are disproportionately more females than males in the compulsive cleaning category, but there is no sex difference in the incidence of checking compulsions. Although the majority of affected people describe some subjective resistance to their compulsions and can recognize its senselessness, the earlier view that these two features (i.e., subjective resistance and recognition of the senselessness of the acts) are universal features of OCD can no longer be supported. Our current knowledge of the nature of abnormal compulsions is derived from psychometric studies, clinical reports, and experimental analysis (cf. Rachman & Hodgson, 1980).

In addition to, or instead of, this subdivision of types of compulsions, problems of this kind can be categorized on a functional basis. The productive functional classification put forward by Mavissakalian (1979) consists of four forms: (a) obsessions; (b) obsessions plus anxiety-reducing compulsions; (c) obsessions plus anxiety-increasing compulsions; and (d) autonomous compulsions. Although some of the therapeutic deductions are open to refinement, this exercise can serve a useful clarifying purpose.

PERSISTENCE

One of the most puzzling aspects of OCD is its persistence. There is no obvious reason for people to engage in repetitive, tiring, embarrassing, and unwanted self-defeating behavior. Nor is there any obvious explanation for the persistent recurrence of intrusive, unacceptable, and distressing thoughts. The persistence of these abnormal experiences and behavior lie at the heart of the matter.

The most favored answer is that compulsive behavior persists precisely because it reduces anxiety. Although this view was proposed in one form or another before the growth of learning theory, it received powerful support from most psychologists who applied learning theory concepts to abnormal behavior. For many years, Mowrer's (1939, 1960) two-stage theory of fear and avoidance, stating that successful avoidance behavior paradoxically preserves fear, was incorporated into many expositions of obsessional-compulsive behavior and has had a profound influence on the way in which we construe these disorders. Although Mowrer's theory served well for a time, some inadequacies have now become apparent (Rachman, 1978), and the theory can no longer provide the basis for a comprehensive account of obsessional compulsive disorders.

It must be said at the outset that the reports given by many OCD patients can be accommodated with ease into the Mowrer view. It is not uncommon for patients to say that they have to carry out their compulsive acts in order to achieve some relief from tension or anxiety. However, this kind of information cannot be conclusive, and there is, moreover, a difficulty from the very source on which one draws—for a small proportion of patients deny that the execution of their compulsive acts is followed by any sense of relief (cf. Beech, 1971,

1974). Fortunately, additional research that has been reported during the past few years has enabled us to achieve some slight advance in our study of these problems. A combination of systematic clinical investigations, psychometric studies, and experimental analyses has put us in a position to draw some fresh and more reliable conclusions about the nature and functions of compulsive acts (cf. Rachman & Hodgson, 1980).

It would appear that most compulsive rituals are indeed followed by a reduction in anxiety/discomfort. This is especially common in the case of cleaning rituals, but there is a small and significant minority of instances (especially in cases of checking rituals) in which the anxiety/discomfort is unaffected by completion of the ritual. In rare cases, anxiety/discomfort increases after the completion of the ritual. Overall, the results are consistent with the anxiety/discomfort-reduction theory, but there are important exceptions. The reduction of anxiety is not a necessary condition for the continuation of compulsive rituals, but it can be a sufficient condition. Although several explanations to account for the persistence of anxiety-elevating obsessions and compulsions have been proposed, none of them appears to be entirely satisfactory. It can be expected, however, that a comprehensive explanation will rest on the recognition of longer term influences that exceed the immediate discomfort produced by executing the compulsion. In other words, the person might be willing to endure a certain amount of discomfort that is produced by carrying out these repetitive rituals in order to ensure that some longer term and more threatening outcome is avoided. The person seeks to reduce the probability of an unwanted but remote event's taking place and is willing, or feels the overpowering need, to carry out repetitive, preventive rituals here and now. The effects of these preventive acts are usually unknowable and hence, are not open to disconfirmation.

If the anxiety/discomfort theory is to survive, it is necessary to demonstrate that in the majority of instances the execution of the appropriate compulsive act is followed by a reduction in anxiety/discomfort. This direct prediction, that the execution of the compulsive activity will be followed by a reduction in anxiety, was the subject of a number of connected experiments by Hodgson and Rachman (1972) and Roper, Rachman, and Hodgson (1973) and Roper and Rachman (1975). A simple experimental procedure was developed that enabled the main predictions to be tested. In the first place, the patients were asked to carry out some activity that would give rise to an increase in anxiety, discomfort, and an accompanying compulsion to carry out the relevant checking or cleaning behavior. Once the anxiety and the associated compulsion were evoked, the patient was asked to carry out the appropriate ritual and report on the strength of his or her compulsive urges and subjective discomfort at each stage. The results of these experiments showed that in the great majority of cases, the completion of the compulsive activity was indeed followed by a reduction in anxiety/discomfort and in the strength of the relevant urge. Among patients with cleaning compulsions, no significant exceptions were encountered. In the case of patients with checking rituals, however, a small number of exceptions occurred in which the completion of the compulsive activity either left the anxiety/discomfort unchanged, or in exceptional circumstances, gave rise to a slight increment in anxiety/discomfort. The general pattern of these results is illustrated in Figure 1.

To begin with, it can be seen that when the person is asked to carry out the appropriate contaminating or disturbing act, he or she immediately experiences a significant increase in anxiety/discomfort and in the associated urge to carry out a cleaning or checking ritual. Having established what

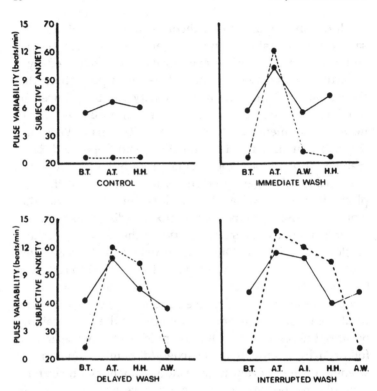

FIGURE 1. Effects of contamination and of cleaning. Results obtained from 12 compulsive cleaners. The mean ratings of anxiety/discomfort (broken line) and of pulse rate variability (solid line), under 4 test conditions, are plotted on the vertical axis. B.T. refers to before touching the contaminant, A.T. means after touching it, A.W. is after washing, H.H. means half-hour, and A.I. means interrupted wash. After touching the contaminant, discomfort showed a large and rapid increase. After washing, there was a large and rapid decrease in discomfort. Neither the mere passage of time (H.H.) nor interruption of the washing (A.I.) had any significant effect on discomfort. From "The Effect of Contamination and Washing in Obsessional Patients" by R. J. Hodgson and S. Rachman, 1972, Behaviour Research & Therapy, 10, p. 113. Copyright 1972. Reprinted by permission.

might be called the *acute* or *active state*, the subjects were asked to carry out the relevant compulsive cleaning or checking activity immediately on instruction, or on other occasions, to carry out their compulsion only after a delay of half an hour. In the case of patients with compulsive cleaning rituals, the relationships were straightforward. Execution of the compulsive cleaning act was rapidly followed by a steep decline in anxiety/discomfort and compulsive urges. In the case of checking rituals, however, the relationship was less clear, and indeed some exceptions occurred.

In the course of these experiments, it was also ascertained that the interruption of a checking or cleaning compulsion was not, as had been expected, followed by an exacerbation of mood state. Rather, the interruption left the level of anxiety/discomfort unaltered. Evidence was also obtained to support the notion that checking rituals, in particular, are muted in the presence of another person but are not fundamentally altered. This finding is in keeping with clinical reports suggesting that wherever possible, people who are under the compulsion to carry out checking rituals greatly prefer to do so when they are alone. By contrast, there was little evidence that cleaning compulsions are modified to any significant extent by the presence of another person.

COMPULSIVE URGES

Using the same experimental paradigm, an attempt was made to collect information about the nature and course of compulsive urges. For the purposes of these experiments, compulsive urges were defined as *impelling forces directed toward a goal*, and it was implied that the source of prompting was internal, even if the urge itself was partially evoked by an external event. In a psychological sense, the compulsive urge is the psychological activity that lies between an obsessional thought and the execution of a compulsive act.

As in the experiments on investigating the persistence of the compulsive behavior, each subject was first exposed to a provoking situation that led to a significant increase in both compulsive urges and in subjective discomfort. As before, it was found that such urges and discomfort can be provoked regularly, reliably, and without difficulty. The natural course of these compulsive urges, their relationship to subjective discomfort, and their amenability to artificial curtailment were analyzed in two connected experiments. The results of the first study, carried out on 11 patients, are shown in Figure 2.

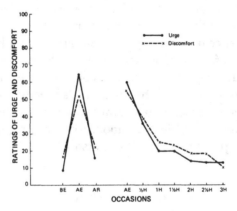

FIGURE 2. The spontaneous decay of compulsive urges. Mean ratings of urge and discomfort reported by 11 compulsive patients. The "natural" decay curve, shown on the right of the figure, is slower and more gradual than seen if the patient carries out his or her ritual (left). On the horizontal axis, B.E. means before exposure, A.E. means after exposure, A.R. means after ritual, and H refers to hour(s). From "The Spontaneous Decay of Compulsive Urges" by S. Rachman, P. de Silva, and G. Roper, 1976, *Behaviour Research & Therapy, 14*, p. 448. Copyright 1976. Reprinted by permission.

With some exceptions, it was found that most patients experienced a marked increase in anxiety/discomfort when exposed to an appropriate provoking situation. Such exposure also produced a marked increase in compulsive urges to carry out the appropriate ritualistic activity. Moreover, execution of the appropriate ritual reduced both discomfort and urges. The reductions were achieved promptly and left only a minimal amount of residual discomfort. It was also possible to trace what can be called the spontaneous decay of compulsive urges. After the urges had been provoked in the experimental situation, a 3-hour observation period was used in order to trace the time course of this so-called spontaneous decay. In most cases, the compulsive urges and associated discomfort underwent a significant decline at the end of the first hour of the observation period, and by 3 hours, at the outside, complete dissipation had occurred. As can be seen from Figure 3A, however, if the person was allowed to carry out the compulsive ritual, this was followed by a rapid and steep decline in compulsive urges. Thus, it is evident that execution of the relevant ritual is functional in the sense that it produces quicker relief. In view of the relative slowness with which compulsive urges and discomfort decay under spontaneous conditions, it is perhaps easy to understand why compulsive rituals develop in the first place. They produce far quicker relief.

Therapeutic experience with OCD patients led us to expect that for many of them the demonstration that they could expect relief from their discomfort and compulsive urges *even* if they refrained from carrying out the relevant ritualistic activity could provide an important learning experience. As a result, we examined the cumulative effects of repeated experiences of such natural spontaneous decays of the compulsive urges and discomfort (Likierman & Rachman, 1980). As had been predicted, the repeated experience of un-dergoing a spontaneous improvement on a number of occasions leads to a lasting decrement in the compulsive urges and discomfort (see Figure 3B).

The four patients who took part in this investigation were all severely disturbed, and the level of their initial discomfort was considerably greater than that observed in the original sample. Probably for this reason, the spontaneous decay

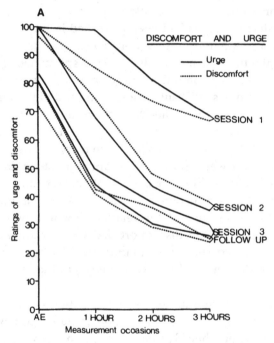

FIGURE 3. The spontaneous decay of compulsive urges: cumulative effects. (A) shows the mean ratings of strength of urge to carry out the ritual ($n = 4$). On the first occasion a gradual decline takes place over 3 hours. However, the decay occurs more quickly on subsequent sessions; now a large measure of decline takes place within 1 hour. The curves suggest that a cumulative process takes place. (B) shows

curve observed on the first day followed a slower path than that described in the first experiment.

The main features of compulsive urges include the following: They can be provoked by external stimulation or, less frequently, arise "spontaneously." Under most conditions, anxiety/discomfort and compulsive urges run parallel courses. Desynchronous changes in this relationship between urges and rituals can occur and are readily provoked by imposing

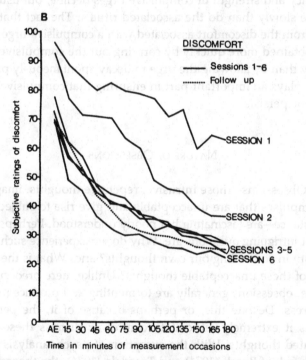

that a similar pattern emerged for ratings of subjective discomfort. From "Spontaneous Decay of Compulsive Urges" by H. Likierman and S. Rachman, 1980, *Behaviour Research & Therapy*,   *18*, p. 389. Copyright 1980. Reprinted by permission.

strict response prevention. Under these conditions, the compulsive acts typically decline earlier than do the compulsive urges. The strength of the compulsive urge usually is related to the strength/frequency of the pertinent compulsive act, that is, they usually covary. Compulsive urges are subject to spontaneous decay, and repeated experiences of such spontaneous decay are followed by a cumulative decline in the strength of the urges. During the course of successful therapy, the frequency and strength of compulsive urges decline, but usually more slowly than do the associated rituals. The fact that relief from the discomfort associated with a compulsive urge can be obtained more quickly by carrying out the compulsive activity than by allowing the urge to decay spontaneously probably plays an important part in ensuring that compulsive behavior persists.

Nature of Obsessions

Obsessions—those intrusive, repetitive thoughts, images, or impulses that are unacceptable and give rise to subjective resistance—are fascinating but poorly understood. Perhaps the most intriguing questions are, Why do we experience such difficulty in controlling our own thoughts? and, What is the origin of these unacceptable thoughts? Unlike mere preoccupations, obsessions generally are tormenting and produce much distress. Despite this, or perhaps because of it, the person finds it extremely difficult to control or dismiss these unwanted thoughts. With the exception of psychoanalysis and the work of Beech (1974) and Teasdale (1974), the theoretical analysis of obsessions has been neglected. There are, of course, methodological obstacles to be overcome before one can come to grips with obsessions, and it is likely that the analysis of obsessions has been delayed by a widespread acceptance of the assumption that they are qualitatively distinct from the cognitive activities of nonpsychiatric subjects. Rachman (1971) conceded that little progress could be expected unless and until it was assumed that most people experience unwanted intrusive thoughts that bear a qualitative similarity to obsessions, even though there are bound to be differences in degree. Starting from this new basis, a research program into the nature of unwanted intrusive thoughts was initiated, and the results will be described later. Before doing so, it is necessary to add some clinical observations on the nature of the obsessions to the definition given previously.

Evidence from clinical surveys indicates that most of these patients are troubled at any particular period by a single dominant obsession. There is a negative correlation between obsessions and slow repetitive rituals. Obsessions tend to be moderately stable, and when the patient has more than one, the obsessions occasionally show shifts in the hierarchy of dominance. People affected by obsessions engage in a wide range of behavior that can be interpreted as escape and avoidance behavior, and this includes not only the obvious forms of avoidance but also covert neutralizing types of behaviors and repeated requests for reassurance. Most of these attempts to deal with obsessional activity can be regarded as equivalent to overt compulsive rituals. Experimental evidence shows that, although the majority of naturally occurring obsessions appear to be generated internally, obsessions can be provoked promptly and with ease (Likierman & Rachman, 1981). They are responsive to, and partly under the control of, external stimulation. The emergence of obsessions produces subjective distress and serious interference with concentration. Like compulsive urges, the emergence of obsessions is associated with the subjective distress and psychophysiological disturbances.

Given certain predisposing factors, intrusive immovable unwanted thoughts are generated by stress and/or mood disturbances. Specific thoughts, images, or impulses can be initiated by external precipitants (e.g., sharp objects) or arise without reference to any detectable trigger. Obsessions take on the properties of noxious stimuli and may in turn contribute to a further deterioration in mood and an increase in sensitivity to stress. Obsessions persist because of the continuing failure of cognitive control coupled with an undue resistance of the obsessional material to normal patterns of habituation. In attempting to achieve relief from his or her discomfort, the affected person engages in avoidance behavior. This kind of activity often is successful in achieving a temporary release from discomfort, but the avoidance behavior is thereby strengthened and may develop compulsive properties. Reviews of the experimental research and clinical surveys have been given by Rachman and Hodgson (1980).

An important source of information about the nature of intrusive unwanted thoughts comes from research by Horowitz (1975) and his colleagues. Using a simple experimental paradigm, in which selected groups of subjects were exposed to stressful visual material, Horowitz was able to gather some valuable new information.

> The results support the hypothesis, based on clinical observation, that persons tend to experience intrusive and stimulus repetitive thoughts after a stress event. . . . The tendency to intrusive and repetitive thought is general in that it occurred in a large proportion of populations not designated as psychiatric patients; and it is general in that it occurs even after the comparatively mild or moderate stress of witnessing an unpleasant film. In other words, compulsive repetitions are not restricted to major stresses or traumas but occur in milder forms after lesser degrees of stress. (Horowitz, 1975, p. 1461)

Building on this foundation, Parkinson and Rachman (1980) were able to confirm the major findings in a study carried out on a group of mothers who were enduring an uncontrived stressful and frightening experience. Among a group of mothers whose children were being admitted to hospital for elective surgery, a steep increase in unwanted intrusive and distressing thoughts was found to occur. Interestingly and reassuringly, this increase in adverse cognitions returned to normal levels very quickly after the successful completion of the operation.

It can be argued that the investigation of intrusive unwanted thoughts is of such intrinsic interest that it requires no further justification. This is my view, but, in any event, we now have grounds for supposing that there is an important connection between intrusive unwanted cognitions and clinical obsessions. Rachman and de Silva (1978) carried out a survey of 124 nonclinical subjects and 8 OCD patients with a view to determining the similarities and differences between clinical obsession and unwanted intrusive thoughts. Their findings were substantially replicated in a second study carried out in 1980 by Parkinson and Rachman. Obsessions in the form of thoughts, images, or impulses certainly are a common experience. A large majority of the respondents reported having experienced unwanted intrusive thoughts of a kind that bear strong similarity to obsessions. It is unknown why a small minority of subjects failed to experience this obsession-allike activity. The form and the content of obsessions reported by nonclinical respondents and by obsessional patients are similar. So-called normal obsessions are also similar to clinical obsessions in their expressed relation to mood and in their meaningfulness to the respondent.

Despite these important similarities of form and content,

normal and abnormal obsessions were found to differ in a number of respects. The threshold of acceptability is higher for abnormal obsessions, which last longer overall and are more vivid than normal obsessions. The abnormal obsessions produce more discomfort, are more frequent, more ego alien, and more strongly resisted than are the normal obsessions. Normal obsessions are easier to dismiss. During the course of these investigations, it was discovered incidentally that most obsessional patients can form the obsession to instruction easily—indeed, they appear better able to do this than nonclinical subjects.

This is not the occasion on which to delve into the deeper nature and significance of normal and abnormal obsessions, but it must be said that if the similarity between these two types of phenomena is accepted, then the attack on clinical obsessions necessarily takes a different form. The questions that quickly arise for consideration are why the abnormal obsessions are so distressing, so prolonged, and so difficult to control. Unfortunately, no satisfactory answer is yet available, but it appears that there is a close association between the amount of distress produced by the obsession and one's inability to control it. It is precisely the distressing obsessions that we find hardest to dismiss. Characteristically, the normal obsessions reported by nonpsychiatric subjects can be dismissed, blocked or diverted, with relatively little effort or difficulty.

So, it would seem that, for some reason, the distressing quality of the obsession impairs our ability to control it. We also have good reason for believing that a person's ability to control or dismiss an unwanted thought, such as an abnormal obsession, is adversely affected by dysphoria. This connection is based on clinical observation (see Rachman & Hodgson, 1980) and so far to a limited extent by experimental analyses. For example, Sutherland, Newman, and Rachman

(1982) found a significant correlation between the time taken to dismiss an intrusive unwanted thought and dysphoria. Transient moods of elation or dysphoria were experimentally induced in nonclinical subjects, who were then asked to obtain and dismiss preselected intrusive thoughts. During the dysphoric mood states, the subjects took longer to remove the thoughts. A satisfactory explanation of the connection between dysphoria and impaired control of intrusive thoughts can be expected to be of theoretical and practical value.

TREATMENT

The pessimism that permeates the psychiatric literature of OCD is nowhere more evident than in discussions regarding outcome. Most writers simply discount the possibility that the outcome can be influenced by treatment. The outcome statistics usually are presented without reference to treatment, and instead, the evidence is discussed, regardless of the type or duration of treatment provided, despite the fact that few patients fail to receive some form of treatment. There is so little confidence in conventional treatment that few writers take the trouble to distinguish between spontaneous remission rates and treatment remission rates. Similarly, most discussions of the prognosis of the disorder contain no mention of the possible influence of formal treatment (e.g., Kringlen, 1970; Lewis, 1966; Lo, 1967). Grimshaw (1964) conducted a useful retrospective study of 100 obsessional patients, followed for a mean of 5 years. He found that roughly two-thirds were improved as far as their symptoms were concerned, and approximately 40% had shown "very considerable improvement." However, he noted that "improvement could not be attributed to a definite form of treatment" (p. 1055). His conclusion was in agreement with the views of most other writers on the subject. In Grimshaw's review, as in others, the proportion of improved cases was not different in any of the major treatment groups. In fact, "the group receiving no specialist treatment fared the best of all, with about 70% having a satisfactory result" (p. 1055). In a wider review covering 13 studies, Goodwin *et al.* (1969) concluded that obsessional neurosis is a chronic illness for which there is no specific treatment. A later, comprehensive review by Black (1974), ended with the conclusion that "no treatment has been shown to influence long-term outcome of obsessional illness...the influence of different therapies can be discounted"(p. 43).

Accurate information on the spontaneous remission rate for this type of disorder is not available, but Cawley (1974) succinctly summarized the position. Among patients with OCD that are severe enough to require admission to hospital, roughly one-quarter will have recovered within 5 years. About one-half will have improved a good deal, and the remaining one-quarter will be unchanged or be worse. For patients whose problems are not sufficiently severe to require admission, roughly two-thirds will be improved to some extent, whereas the remaining third will have shown slight improvement or remain unchanged or become worse. Further consideration of spontaneous remission rates in this and related disorders is given by Rachman and Wilson (1980). In view of the occurrence of spontaneous remission—a fact of considerable importance to practicing clinicians and their patients—it is essential that the claims made on behalf of any form of treatment should be evaluated against the naturally occurring remission rate.

In the use of medication for OCD, this type of controlled evaluation has infrequently been carried out, and therefore one has to regard the claims made on behalf of various drugs with some caution. A full review is given by Ananth in Chapter 5. On present evidence, the types of drugs most worthy of consideration as possible therapeutic agents in coping with OCD are the so-called antidepressants. Given the close association between depression and OCD it is reasonable to expect that any successful antidepressant treatment, using drugs or other means, should be capable of producing useful changes in many cases. The antidepressant drug that has attracted most attention so far is clomipramine. This drug has achieved some popularity not only because of its satisfactorily demonstrated effects on depression, but also because it has been claimed that the drug has a specific therapeutic effect on obsessional-compulsive symptoms (e.g. Fernandez & Lopez-Ibor, 1969) and Capstick (1973), among others. Rachman *et al.*(1979) carried out a randomized control trial on 40 moderately to severely disabled OCD patients, focusing primarily on the effects of behavioral treatment, but including clomipramine. For present purposes, it is sufficient to remark that convincing evidence was obtained that clomipramine had a primary therapeutic effect on depression and a secondary effect on obsessional problems. Among those patients who were not unduly troubled by depression prior to the administration of the drug, there were few signs of any improvement in obsessional-compulsive problems as a consequence of taking clomipramine. On the other hand, there was good evidence that among those patients who were suffering from at least moderate levels of depression as well as obsessional problems, the successful use of the antidepressant drug was, on the whole, followed by significant improvement in some of the obsessional difficulties. In their study, Thoren *et al.* (1980) obtained supporting evidence of the therapeutic value of clomipramine, with a response rate of "about 50%" (p. 1285). The evidence of a direct effect on obsessional-compulsive symptoms was conflicting and not evident on the patients' reports of their symptoms or on ratings of daily tasks. The beneficial effects of the drug were maintained only during drug administration. Relapses on withdrawal were quickly evident.

The important question of whether or not clomipramine has a specific antiobsessional action in addition to its antidepressant effects is best attacked by a direct prospective comparison between depressed and nondepressed patients matched for severity and duration of disorder. The results of this comparison, valuable in their own right, should also increase our understanding of the relations between depression and obsessional-compulsive disorders. We are poised on the edge of a significant advance in understanding.

Although some ambitious claims have been made on behalf of the therapeutic power of interpretive psychotherapy, Cawley (1974) concluded his review of the evidence by saying that "there is no evidence to support or refute the proposition that formal psychotherapy helps patients with obsessional disorders" (p. 288). His conclusion that these disorders are unlikely to be helped by formal psychotherapy appears to be shared by a majority of writers, excluding those, of course, who are proponents of the psychoanalytic method. An exception is Malan, a prominent clinician and researcher at the Tavistock Clinic, the leading psychoanalytic institution in Britain. "It is apparently true for instance, that there is no known authenticated case of an obsessive hand-washer being cured by psychoanalytic treatment" (Malan, 1979, pp. 218–219). A wide-ranging review of the effects of psychotherapy has been provided by Rachman and Wilson (1980).

For a period lasting approximately 15 years, psychosurgery was a commonly used form of treatment for obsessional problems, particularly those of a seemingly intractable character. In view of the seriousness of these operations and the fact they are still in use, albeit on a greatly reduced scale, a more comprehensive examination of the evidence on this subject appears to be warranted (Rachman, 1979).

The belief that psychosurgery is an effective method of treating OCD rests on two main claims. In the first place, it is argued that psychosurgery is particularly suitable for treating such disorders, and secondly, it is claimed to be the only effective method of treating the most severe and intractable cases. If sustained, these claims would be of considerable importance, offering as they do some hope for those patients who, by definition, are beyond help by other methods.

Before examining the evidence on the effects of psychosurgery, it is well to recall that these operations were initially introduced as a cure, not for obsessions, but for schizophrenia. Predictably, the use of surgery was soon extended to include a wide range of disorders from depression to delinquency (Rachman, 1979). As the skepticism about the value of psychosurgery as a treatment for schizophrenia grew, a shift of emphasis occurred and more and more obsessional patients received the operation. It need hardly be argued that the use of radical surgical procedures can only be justified on grounds of demonstrable success in the absence of satisfactory alternatives.

The first reason for misgivings is that no serious attempt has ever been made to explain why psychosurgery *should* alleviate obsessional disorders; even if we possessed acceptable empirical proof of its therapeutic value, we would remain in the dark about the causal processes involved. The earlier but now discredited claim that psychosurgery is an effective treatment for schizophrenia is doubly troublesome. It reminds us of our credulity in therapeutic matters and also reminds us that the recommendation of surgery for OCD is secondhand

and atheoretical. It is also worth bearing in mind that use of surgery is based upon, and helps to, perpetuate the dubious notion that all OCDs are illnesses. There can be little doubt that acceptance of the alternative view, that OCD is better construed as a psychological problem (cf. Rachman & Hodgson, 1980), would reduce the likelihood of anyone recommending a surgical solution.

An extensive review of the major reports on the effects of psychosurgery has been given in Rachman (1979), and the present account is confined to the most recent and major studies. Smith, Kiloh, Cochrane, and Klijajic (1976) evaluated the effects of leucotomy on 43 patients, including 5 obsessional cases. Three of their patients died, 3 developed adverse personality changes, and 1 had repeated seizures. At the 6-month follow-up, 58% of the patients were said to be markedly improved, but the obsessional patients did slightly less well than others. Among these patients, the improvement was only slight to moderate. The best results in this series appear to have been achieved by the depressed patients, a not uncommon finding (cf. Rachman, 1979). As the Smith study meets few of the criteria generally regarded as being necessary for controlled studies, this partial evidence cannot be given much weight. The comparatively favorable reports by Sykes and Tredgold (1964) and by Strom-Olsen and Carlisle (1971) cannot be ignored, but, as both these reports are retrospective, nonrandom, uncontrolled, and based on a partial sample of patients, firm conclusions cannot be reached. On the question of whether or not the operation is best reserved for the most intractable cases, the information that in the Strom-Olsen series 4 out of the 20 patients were operated on after a duration of illness of less than 5 years is a disturbing feature. The operation is not, in practice, reserved for chronic or intractable disorders.

Kelly *et al.* (1972) reported a favorable improvement rate of 90% for the 40 patients who were included in their prospective noncontrolled study. Seventeen of the 40 patients had a diagnosis of obsessional neurosis. Although cured or much improved outcomes were reported for 7 out of the 17 patients, by counting the 6 patients who fell into the center of the rating scale, Kelly, Walter, Mitchell-Heggs, and Sargant (1972) were able to quote an improvement rate of 76% for the obsessional subsample. This optimistic picture, however, must be seen against the similar claim of a 66% improvement rate for most of their patients who were diagnosed as schizophrenic—a very unusual result.

These almost entirely favorable results, observed 6 weeks after the operation, should be regarded with caution as the study suffers from the defects of rater contamination, confounded treatments, absence of a control, and so on. A follow-up report on this study has been given by Mitchell-Heggs, Kelly, and Richardson (1976).

Their impressive follow-up data should not obscure the original defects of the study. It should also be mentioned that the ages of the patients, at the time of the operation, ranged from 21 to 65 years. The lower limit confirms that the operation is not reserved for chronic cases. Furthermore, roughly 12% had an illness duration of less than 5 years. Even if one sets aside the flaws in the design of the study, the reasons for the apparent improvement are unknown. The explanations that are offered, and all of these are tentative, suggest that the reductions in obsessional-compulsive problems that might have occurred are bound to be *secondary*. But if this is granted, then it must be demonstrated that the *primary* action, be it the relief of anxiety or the reduction of depression, cannot be achieved by easier and nonintrusive means. Even if their astonishing claim of an 80% success rate for the schizophrenic patients gives rise for considerable caution, their claims at least establish that psychosurgery might be worth investigation if a plausible rationale can be offered and if there is no alternative form of therapy available. On a broader view, however, it can be argued, as I do, that psychosurgery is a redundant and undesirable treatment and that there are preferable alternatives.

Bridges, Goktepe, and Maratos (1973) carried out a retrospective follow-up study of 24 OCD patients and 24 depressive patients who had undergone psychosurgery at least 3 years earlier. Although the information on the status of the patients was gathered in a direct and methodical manner, the absence of any preoperative information is a serious shortcoming. For what it is worth, however, the depressed patients in this retrospective survey did as well as, or slightly better than, the OCD patients. This result serves to emphasize the point made earlier that whatever else it is, psychosurgery of this kind is not a *specific* remedy for OCD. Furthermore, evidence of serious unwanted effects was uncovered in the Bridges survey (e.g., 5 of the 48 patients suffered fits after the operation; 10 of the 48 patients had to have more than one operation, etc.).

In regard to the common claim that psychosurgery is particularly effective for chronic intractable cases, the obsessional patients who did worst in this retrospective survey had an illness duration of 13 years and those who did best had an illness duration of 9 years. Those patients who had the longest admissions to hospital prior to the operation did worst of all. In a later and more extensive review, Goktepe, Young, and Bridges (1975) found a similar pattern among a larger sample of patients. As in most of these reports, the depressive patients appeared to have done best. So, even if the evidence were interpreted, with minimal caution, as showing that psychosurgery benefits a proportion of OCD patients, it certainly cannot be concluded that surgery is particularly suitable for managing this type of neurosis. Finally, both Cawley (1974) and Sternberg (1974) concluded that those patients who have a better prognosis without psychosurgery are precisely the ones who are said to respond well to the operation. In Ingram's (1961) summary, he stated that "many of the factors said to favour the outcome of the operation are seen to be the same as those favouring spontaneous improvement" (p. 399).

To return to the opening question of this section, it must be concluded that on present evidence, neither of the therapeutic claims made on behalf of psychosurgery is supportable. Psychosurgery is not particularly suitable for treating obsessional disorders, and it is not most effective for treating chronic or intractable cases. Proponents of psychosurgery justify its use on empirical grounds, but it turns out that this empirically based treatment has an inadequate empirical basis. In the present circumstances, there is little reason to recommend psychosurgery for obsessional disorders.

It should be borne in mind that the resort to psychosurgery often was an act of desperation on the part of clinicians whose therapeutic efforts all too often proved to be powerless. With psychosurgery as the last, or all but last, procedure available to clinicians, it can be seen how very important it was and is to find acceptable alternatives. In fact, the looming threat of surgery for neurotic patients acted as a spur to behavioral psychologists on a number of occasions. There can be little doubt that as the power and range of behavioral and other psychological methods for dealing with OCD increase, we shall see the last of psychosurgery as a method for dealing with these difficulties. There is a good deal to be said for reminding oneself, and others, that for a period of nearly 20 years, behavioral methods of treating OCD were in active competition with psychosurgery.

As Foa will provide a full evaluation of the effects of behavioral therapy (see Chapter 2), these observations will be summarily brief. It is generally agreed that the first successes achieved by behavior therapists dealing with neuroses came in the modification of phobias. Wolpe's (1958, 1973) invaluable pioneering work has been consolidated by the addition of new information and the development of refined and novel techniques (see Rachman, 1978). Among these new techniques, flooding and participant modeling are among the most promising. Unfortunately, the early successes achieved in the treatment of phobias were not accompanied by the same progress in dealing with obsessional disorders. Until recently, therapists approached the treatment of obsessional disorders with realistic caution. Even when the traditional fear-reducing method of desensitization was successfully used, the treatment turned out to be laborious and time consuming. The position prevailing at the end of the 1960s has been summarized in a review by Meyer, Levy, and Schnurer (1974). They concluded that the success rates reported by behavior therapists dealing with OCD were significantly lower than those achieved in working with other disorders. They collected clinical reports on the treatment of 61 obsessional patients, and the overall success rate was discouraging. Moreover, they noted that a surprisingly large number of treatment variations had been attempted and this is seldom a good sign.

The medley of predominantly imaginal methods that were tried on OCD patients during the 1960s gradually gave way to *in vivo* methods of treatment with modeling, exposure and response-prevention techniques taking places of major importance. By the early 1970s, a significant change had occurred, and then, for many people suffering from OCD, participation in a program of behavioral treatment helped them achieve substantial relief and benefits. This advance occurred as a result of a combination of several events and influences.

In the first place, there was a shift in emphasis in treatment programs provided for phobic patients, from a reliance on imaginal presentations to *in vivo* exposures. This change in emphasis, in turn, was influenced by claims that implosion was capable of producing large and rapid clinical improvements. At approximately the same time and for some common reasons, research workers began to show renewed interest in the therapeutic possibilities of *flooding*, defined concisely as relatively prolonged exposures to high-intensity stimulation. This interest was boosted by the methodical and helpful research carried out on animals by Baum (1970). He was able to demonstrate that the technique of response prevention was capable of reducing intense avoidance behavior in a relatively short time. Soon, attempts were being made to reduce people's fears by exposing them to intense stimulation for prolonged periods while discouraging their attempts at escape. Bandura's (1969) brilliant revival of the concept of *imitation* and his development of *social learning theory* (see Bandura, 1977) were soon followed by the appearance of therapuetic modeling procedures. Therapeutic modeling was one of the first methods ever to produce a result that exceeded the fear-reducing effects of desensitization (Bandura, Gruset, & Menlove, 1967). Like flooding, therapeutic modeling is almost always carried out *in vivo*.

Bearing in mind the now-evident similarities between phobias and certain types of OCDs, notably those involving predominantly cleaning rituals, it was inevitable that these new fear-reducing techniques would be recruited in a fresh attack on unyielding compulsions and obsessions. Therapists also drew valuable encouragement and advice from Meyer's (1966) extremely instructive account of his success in treating two seriously handicapped patients. He regarded the favorable outcome in these two cases as being the result of a successful attempt to modify the patients' expectations. He also laid emphasis on the need for the treatment to "be intensive" and "to have a strict control over the patient's behaviour" (p. 280). While engaged in research into the fear-reducing mechanisms involved in flooding and in Stampfl's implosion method, Hodgson and Rachman decided to test the value of these methods during the course of their protracted attempts to help three severely disabled obsessional-compulsive patients. The development of this work, with its disappointments and successes, has been recounted by Rachman and Hodgson (1980). For present purposes, it is sufficient to say that we were encouraged in our belief that modeling exposure and response prevention might prove to be a sufficiently powerful combination to modify even such an unyielding disorder as OCD. As a result, a connected series of clinical trials was undertaken in collaboration with Roper, Marks, Sartory, Grey, McDonald, and a number of other colleagues. (These results are discussed by Foa in Chapter 2.) Taken in conjunction with the other research findings, some conclusions are merited.

The combination of exposure and response prevention is a powerful and reliable method for producing changes, especially in compulsive behavior. It seems improbable that response prevention acting alone is that unless the person is in those cases that are predominantly of the checking variety. The reason for having reservations about the value of response prevention's acting alone is that unless the person is being exposed to the provoking stimulation, the prevention of compulsive responses is likely to be empty. Stated plainly, there has to be a *response* to *prevent*. It would be meaningless to ask compulsive hand washers to refrain from washing their hands unless they are already in a contaminated state.

How important is the therapeutic contribution of exposure? It would appear that although exposure alone may be sufficient (but not essential—see de Silva & Rachman, 1981) in some instances a failure to institute response-prevention procedures might well undermine the otherwise beneficial effects of exposure. In cases where there is a strong phobic element, repeated exposures can be expected to achieve much, regardless of response prevention. In checking compulsions, however, failure to institute response prevention is likely to end in therapeutic failure. The components of treatment are analyzed by Foa in Chapter 2.

Turning to the less common forms of OCD, it has to be admitted that at present we are inadequately prepared for dealing with primary obsessional slowness or pure obsessions. Until we are in possession of information gathered from properly conducted controlled trials, the following guidelines are offered in the hope that they might be of value to therapists. Patients suffering from primary obsessional slowness appear to respond well to a program based on modeling and target-setting therapeutic instructions (Rachman & Hodgson, 1980). Once an appropriate program incorporating a ladder of targets is constructed, the therapist provides modeling for the patient. Thereafter, the patient's progress is monitored in a way that enables both therapist and patient to overcome obstacles as they arise. These programs generally require much domiciliary practice.

Obsessions, pure but seldom simple, are a far more puzzling phenomenon than primary obsessional slowness, and at present we have an insecure grasp of their nature (Rachman, 1978). In cases of pure obsessions, uncomplicated by overt compulsive acts, at present the best approach would appear to be habituation training carried out under relaxation and/or the evocation of the thoughts to therapeutic instruction. Where the obsessions are followed by internal or external neutralizing activities, these should be put under response-prevention instructions. Further advice on this subject must await the outcome of current research programs (cf. Likierman & Rachman, 1981).

Summary

The concept of obsessional-compulsive disorders is well established and denotes behavior and experiences that are easily recognized in almost all cases. Obsessions are repeatedly experienced, unwanted, intrusive thoughts/images/impulses, the contents of which are usually repugnant to the person who is experiencing them. Compulsive behavior is repetitive, stereotyped behavior that is preceded or accompanied by strong urges to carry out the behavior despite its acknowledged irrational features. Most but not all obsessions and compulsions are met with internal resistance. The most common types of compulsive behaviors are repetitive cleaning or checking behavior. People who have OCD generally experience both obsessions and compulsions, but in a significant minority of cases, obsessions only are experienced. Obsessional-compulsive disorders are not common, but they tend to be more serious and enduring than other forms of neurosis.

The disorders generally emerge in early adulthood, are closely associated with affective disorders, often take a fluctuating course in the early stages, and have roughly a one-in-three chance of becoming chronic problems.

There is a close relationship between OCD and depression, but this is not invariant. Close connections between OCD and phobias are also common, particularly in cases of cleaning compulsions. There is little certainty about the conditions that promote the disorders, but evidence of genetic and social transmission has been gathered. The genetic factors are likely to be general and the social or personal influences more specific in their effects. In a large minority of cases, particularly those in which cleaning compulsions are prominent, a precipitating event can be traced. On the whole, checking compulsions develop more gradually and are less often associated with a specific onset.

It seems probable that in most instances, compulsive behavior is maintained because it generally is followed by a reduction in anxiety/discomfort. The maintaining conditions of obsessional activities are poorly understood, but the distressing qualities of the unwanted cognitions and the presence of dysphoria are two factors that seem to impair one's ability to control and dismiss unwanted cognitions.

Until the 1970s, little could be done to improve on the spontaneous remission rate of OCD, which was roughly estimated to be lower than 60% within 2 years of onset. The introduction of antidepressant medication has produced promising results, but at present the best established method is exposure and response prevention—a behavioral technique of demonstrated effectiveness in reducing compulsive behavior. Although useful theoretical advances have been made, reliable methods for modifying obsessions have yet to be demonstrated. As far as obsessional-compulsive disorders generally are concerned, there are grounds for anticipating that some significant advances in our understanding will occur in the near future.

REFERENCES

Akhtar, S., Wig, N. H., Verma, V. K., Pershod, D., & Verma, S. K. A phenomenological analysis of symptoms in obsessive-compulsive neuroses. *British Journal of Psychiatry*, 1975, *127*, 342–348.

Bandura, A. *The principles of behavior modification.* New York: Holt, Rinehart & Winston, 1969.

Bandura, A. *Social learning theory.* Prentice-Hall. Englewood Cliffs, NJ

Bandura, A., Grusec, J., and Menlove, F. Vicarious extinction of avoidance behavior. *Journal of Personality and Social Psychology,* 1967, 5, 449–455.

Baum, M. Extinction of avoidance responding through response prevention (flooding). *Psychological Bulletin,* 1970, 74, 276.

Beech, H. R. Ritualistic activity in obsessional patients. *Journal of Psychosomatic Research,* 1971, 15, 417–422.

Beech, H. R. (Ed.). *Obsessional states.* London: Methuen, 1974.

Birley, J. Modified frontal leucotomy: A review of 106 cases. *British Journal of Psychiatry,* 1964, 110, 211–221.

Black, A. The natural history of obsessional neurosis. In H. R. Beech (Ed.), *Obsessional states.* London: Methuen, 1974.

Bridges, P., Goktepe, E., & Maratos, J. A comparative review of patients with obsessional neurosis and with depression treated by psychosurgery. *British Journal of Psychiatry,* 1973, 123, 663–674.

Capstick, N. Clomipramine in the treatment of true obsessional state—A report on four patients. *Psychosomatics,* 1973, 16(1), 21–25.

Carey, G. *A clinical genetic study of obsessional and phobic states.* Unpublished doctoral dissertation, University of Minnesota, 1978. Quoted by Murray et al. (1981).

Carr, A. Compulsive neurosis: A review of the literature. *Psychological Bulletin,* 1974, 81, 311–318.

Cawley, R. H. Psychotherapy and obsessional disorders. In H. R. Beech (Ed.), *Obsessional states.* London: Methuen, 1974.

de Silva, P., & Rachman, S. Is exposure a necessary condition for fear-reduction? *Behaviour Research & Therapy,* 1981, 19, 227–232.

Eysenck, H. J., & Rachman, S. *The causes and cures of neurosis.* London: Routledge & Kegan Paul, 1965.

Fernandez, R. & Lopez-Ibor, R. Mono-chlorimipramine in the treatment of psychiatric patients. *Acta Esperimentale Neurologia,* 1969, 26, 119–147.

Gittelson, N. The fate of obsessions in depressive psychosis. *British Journal of Psychiatry,* 1966, 112, 705–708.

Goktepe, E., Young, L., & Bridges, P. A further review of the results of stereotactic subcaudate/tractotomy. *British Journal of Psychiatry,* 1975, 126, 270–280.

Goodwin, D., Guze, S., & Robins, E. Follow-up studies in obsessional neurosis. *Archives of General,* 1969, 20, 182–187.

Grimshaw, L. Obsessional disorder and neurological illness. *Journal of Neurology, Neurosurgery and Psychiatry,* 1964, 27, 229–231.

Hare, E., Price, J., & Slater, E. Fertility in obsessional neurosis. *British Journal of Psychiatry,* 1972, 121, 197–205.

Hodgson, R. J., & Rachman, S. The effects of contamination and washing in obsessional patients. *Behaviour Research & Therapy*, 1972, 10, 111–117.

Horowitz, M. Intrusive and repetitive thoughts after experimental stress. *Archives of General Psychiatry*, 1975, 32, 1457–1463.

Ingram, I. M. Obsessional illness in mental hospital patients. *Journal of Mental Science*, 1961, 197, 382–402.

Inouye, E. Similar and dissimilar manifestations of obsessive-compulsive neurosis in monozygotic twins. *American Journal Psychiatry*, 1965, 121, 1171–1175.

Jaspers, K. *General psychopathology*. Chicago: University of Chicago Press, 1963.

Kelly, D., Walter, C., Mitchell-Heggs, N., & Sargant, W. Modified leucotomy assessed clinically, physiologically and psychologically at six weeks and eighteen months. *British Journal of Psychiatry*, 1972, 120, 19.

Kringlen, E. Obsessional neurotics: A long-term follow-up. *British Journal of Psychiatry*, 1965, 111, 709–722.

Kringlen, E. Natural history of obsessional neurosis. *Seminars in Psychiatry*, 1970, 2, 403–419.

Lewis, A. Problems of obsessional illness. *Proceedings of the Royal Society of Medicine*, 1936, 29, 325–336.

Lewis, A. Obsessional disorder. In R. Scott (Ed.), *Price's textbook of the practice of medicine* (10th ed.). London: Oxford University Press, 1966.

Likierman, H., & Rachman, S. Spontaneous decay of compulsive urges. *Behaviour Research & Therapy*, 1980, 18, 387–394.

Likierman, H., & Rachman, S. Obsessions: An experimental investigation of thought stopping and habituation training. *Behavioral Psychotherapy*, 1982, 10, 324–328.

Lo, W. A follow-up study of obsessional neurotics in Hong Kong Chinese. *British Journal of Psychiatry*, 1967, 113, 823–832.

Malan, D. *Individual psychotherapy and the science of psychodynamics*. London: Butterworths, 1979.

Mavissakalian, M. Functional classification of obsessive-compulsive phenomena. *Journal of Behavioral Assessment*, 1979, 1, 271–279.

Meyer, V. Modification of expectations in cases with obsessional rituals. *Behaviour Research & Therapy*, 1966, 4, 273–280.

Meyer, V., Levy, R., & Schnurer, A. The behavioral treatment of obsessive-compulsive disorder. In H. R. Beech (ed.), *Obsessional states*. London: Methuen, 1974.

Mitchell-Heggs, N., Kelly, D., & Richardson, A. A stereotactic limbic leucotomy—A follow-up at 16 months. *British Journal of Psychiatry*, 1976, 128, 226–240.

Mowrer, O. H. A stimulus-response theory of anxiety. *Psychological Review*, 1939, 46, 555–565.

Mowrer, O. *Learning theory and behavior*. New York: Wiley, 1960.

Murray, R., Clifford, C., Fulker, D., & Smith, A. Is there a genetic contribution to obsessional traits and symptoms? In M. Tsuang & N. Watson (Eds.), *Genetic issues*. New York: Academic Press, 1981.

Parkinson, L., & Rachman, S. Are intrusive thoughts subject to habituation? *Behaviour Research & Therapy*, 1980, *18*, 409–418.

Pollitt, J. Natural history of obsessional states. *British Medical Journal*, 1957, *1*, 195–198.

Rachman, S. Obsessional ruminations. *Behaviour Research and Therapy*, 1971, *9*, 229–235.

Rachman, S. The modification of obsessions: A new formulation. *Behaviour Research & Therapy*, 1976, *14*, 437–443.

Rachman, S. An anatomy of obsessions. *Behavior Analysis and Modification*, 1978, *2*, 255–278.

Rachman, S. Psychosurgical treatment of obsessional-compulsive disorders. In E. Valenstein (Ed.), *The psychosurgery debate*. San Francisco: W. H. Freeman, 1979.

Rachman, S., & de Silva, P. Abnormal and normal obsessions. *Behaviour Research & Therapy*, 1978, *16*, 233–248.

Rachman, S., & Hodgson, R. *Obsessions and compulsions*. Englewood Cliffs, NJ: Prentice-Hall, 1980.

Rachman, S., & Wilson, G. T. *The effects of psychological therapy*. Oxford: Pergamon Press, 1980.

Rachman, S., Hodgson, R., & Marks, I. The treatment of chronic obsessional neurosis. *Behaviour Research & Therapy*, 1971, *9*, 237–247.

Rachman, S., de Silva, P., & Roper, G. The spontaneous decay of compulsive urges. *Behaviour Research & Therapy*, 1976, *14*, 445–453.

Rachman, S., Cobb, J., MacDonald, B., Mawson, D., Sartory, G., & Stern, R. The behavioral treatment of obsessional-compulsive disorders, with and without clomipramine. *Behaviour Research & Therapy*, 1979, *17*, 467–478.

Roper, G., & Rachman, S. Obsessional-compulsive checking: Replication and development. *Behaviour Research & Therapy*, 1975, *14*, 25–32.

Roper, G., Rachman, S., & Hodgson, R. An experiment on obsessional checking. *Behaviour Research & Therapy*, 1973, *11*, 271–277.

Rosenberg, C. Familial aspects of obsessional neurosis. *British Journal of Psychiatry*, 1967, *113*, 405–413.

Rosenthal, D. *Genetic theory and abnormal behavior*. New York: McGraw-Hill, 1970.

Salzman, L., & Thaler, F. Obsessive-compulsive disorders: A review of the literature. *American Journal of Psychiatry*, 1981, *138*, 286–296.

Shields, J. Heredity and psychological abnormality. In H. J. Eysenck (Ed.), *Handbook of abnormal psychology (2nd ed.)*. London: Pitmans, 1973.

Skoog, G. The anancastic syndrome. *Acta Psychiatrica et Neurologica Scandinavica*, 1959, *34* (Suppl. 134).

Slater, E., & Cowie, V. *The genetics of mental disorders*. London: Oxford University Press, 1971.

Smith, J. S., Kiloh, L. G., Cochrane, N., & Klijajic, I. A prospective evaluation of open prefrontal leucotomy. *Medical Journal of Australia*, 1976, *1*, 731–735.

Stern, R. S., & Cobb, J. Phenomenology of obsessive-compulsive neurosis. *British Journal of Psychiatry*, 1978, *132*, 233–239.

Sternberg, M. Physical treatments in obsessional disorders. In H. R. Beech (Ed.), *Obsessional states*. London: Methuen, 1974.

Strom-Olsen, R., & Carlisle, S. Bi-frontal stereotactic trachotomy. *British Journal of Psychiatry*, 1971, *118*, 141–154.

Sutherland, G., Newman, B., & Rachman, S. Experimental investigations of the relations between mood and intrusive unwanted cognitions. *British Journal of Medical Psychology*, 1982, *55*, 127–128.

Sykes, M., & Tredgold, R. Restricted orbital undercutting. *British Journal of Psychiatry*, 1964, *110*, 609–640.

Teasdale, J. Learning models of obsessional-compulsive disorder. In H. R. Beech (Ed.), *Obsessional states*. London: Methuen, 1974.

Templer, D. I. The obsessive-compulsive neurosis: Review of research findings. *Comprehensive Psychiatry*, 1972, *13*, 375–383.

Thoren, P., Asberg, M., Cronholm, B., Jornestadt, L., & Traskman, L. Clomipramine treatment of obsessive-compulsive disorder. *Archives of General Psychiatry*, 1980, *37*, 1281–1285.

Tienari, P. Psychiatric illnesses in identical twins. *Acta Psyciatrica Scandinavica*, (Suppl. 171), 1963.

Videbech, T. The psychopathology of anacastic endogenous depression. *Acta Psychiatrica Scandinavica*, 1975, *52*, 336–373.

Wilner, A., Reich, T., Robins, I., Fishman, R., & van Doren, T. Obsessive-compulsive neurosis. *Comprehensive Psychiatry*, 1976, *17*, 527–539.

Wolpe, J. *Psychotherapy by reciprocal inhibition*. Stanford: Stanford University Press, 1958.

Wolpe, J. *The practice of behavior therapy* (2nd ed.). Oxford: Pergamon Press, 1973.

2

Behavior Therapy
with Obsessive-Compulsives

FROM THEORY TO TREATMENT

E. B. FOA, G. S. STEKETEE, AND B. J. OZAROW

DEFINITION

Clinical accounts of obsessive-compulsive disorders (OCD) have appeared in the literature for well over 100 years. Esquirol first described this syndrome in 1838, but it was not until the beginning of this century that attempts were made to formally document and define it (Janet, 1903; Lewis, 1935; Schneider, 1925). Traditional conceptualizations of OCD have generally included both cognitive and behavioral components. For example, Pollitt (1956) suggested that this disorder is characterized by

E. B. FOA and G. S. STEKETEE • Temple University, Department of Psychiatry, EPPI, 3300 Henry Avenue, Philadelphia, Pennsylvania 19129. B. J. OZAROW • Department of Psychology, Aquinas College, Grand Rapids, Michigan 49506. Preparation of this chapter was supported by Grant MH 31634 awarded to the first author by the National Institute of Mental Health.

a recurrent or persistent idea, thought, image, feeling, impulse
or movement which is accompanied by a sense of subjective
compulsion and desire to resist it, the event being recognized
by the individual as foreign to his personality and into the abnormality of which he has insight. (p. 842)

Conventional formulations of OCD have typically referred
to thoughts, images, and impulses as obsessions, whereas
repetitive overt actions have been defined as compulsions.
This modality-based distinction poses serious conceptual problems that become apparent when symptoms of specific patients are examined. One patient experienced as much discomfort from physical contact with chicken soup as from the mere
thought of it. He relieved the former discomfort by washing
(overt ritual) and the latter by the thought *Palmolive* (covert,
cognitivie ritual). In a second case, the number 3 provoked
anxiety in the patient whereas the number 7 reduced it. Here
not only are the two manifestations of the same modality, but
they also belong to the same class (both are numbers); yet,
one elicits anxiety, whereas the otehr reduces it. These observations point out the inadequacies of the traditional definitions
and suggest that alternative conceptualizations are needed.

These considerations have led Foa and Tillmanns (1980)
to propose a definition based on the functional relationship between obsessive-compulsive symptoms and anxiety. According to this model, obsessions or ruminations are defined as
thoughts, images, or actions that *generate* anxiety. Compulsions, on the other hand, are conceived of as attempts to alleviate the anxiety aroused by the obsession and take the form
of either overt actions or covert cognitive (neutralizing) events.
As noted by Rachman (1976a), these two types of responses
are functionally equivalent.

Thus, we suggest that the obsessive-compulsive syndrome
consists of a set of events (overt or covert) that are anxiety

evoking; these are labeled *obsessions*. To alleviate anxiety evoked by the obsessions, a set of behaviors (overt or covert) are performed; these are called *compulsions*. This definition is consistent with the behavioral model of obsessive-compulsive disorders and the treatment interventions that have been derived from this model.

BEHAVIORAL MODELS

Mowrer's Two-Stage Theory

A widely accepted model for conceptualizing the acquisition and maintenance of obsessive-compulsive symptoms is the two-stage theory of fear and avoidance first proposed by Mowrer (1939) and later elaborated by Dollard and Miller (1950). According to this theory, the learning of fear and avoidance involves two distinct stages. In the first stage, a neutral stimulus acquires anxiety-evoking properties by being paired with an unconditional stimulus (classical conditioning). Next, because of the aversive properties of the stimulus, escape and/or avoidance responses are developed. These reponses are subsequently reinforced through their ability to reduce anxiety (negative reinforcement). Higher order conditioning occurs when the organism associates other neutral stimuli (such as words, images, or thoughts, as well as concrete objects) with the initial conditioned stimulus. Because of this process, the original conditioning is often obscured, and the associated anxiety is diffused into a general feeling of discomfort.

In obsessive-compulsives, the escape or avoidance responses take the form of ritualistic/compulsive behaviors and are maintained by the consequent reduction of anxiety (Dollard & Miller, 1950). A similar process of negative reinforcement also appears to take place in phobic patients. Despite the presence of this common feature, the two disorders differ in a number of important respects. One such difference centers around the fact that escape behaviors of phobic patients are clearly related to the feared object. For example, height phobics organize their lives to avoid being in high places. By contrast, the relationship between specific compulsions and the eliciting stimuli may not be so clear. Some rituals are logically related to the source of anxiety. For instance, praying may reduce the fear of having committed a mortal sin, and mentally enumerating the day's events may offset the chance that something important will be forgotten. Other rituals seem to be acquired by chance; when first performed in the presence of the evoking stimuli, they may have produced relief and are then repeated whenever the discomfort-arousing stimuli are present. The more patients engage in "relief-producing behavior," the more convinced they become that only this specific behavior can offset their discomfort.

A further difference between phobics and obsessive-compulsives stems from the fact that phobic stimuli can often be successfully avoided, so that no confrontation occurs. But intrusive, disturbing thoughts are less easily escaped. Additionally, the high degree of generalization and the higher order conditioning that takes place in obsessive-compulsive disorders progressively decreases the effectiveness of mere avoidance of those external stimul that give rise to obsessions. Eventually, there are just too many stimuli to be avoided. Specific behavior patterns are then developed to terminate or reduce discomfort. These "active" avoidance patterns, as opposed to the "passive" ones of phobics, are often stereotyped and performed in a rigid manner and are thus referred to as rituals or compulsions.

Although there has been some controversy regarding the anxiety-reducing effect of rituals (Beech, 1971), there is significant research supporting the drive reduction theory. Using physiological and subjective indices of anxiety, several studies have reported decreased anxiety following performance of overt rituals (Carr, 1971; Hodgson & Rachman, 1972; Hornsveld, Kraaimaat, & van Dam-Baggen, 1979; Roper & Rachman, 1976; Roper, Rachman, & Hodgson, 1973). Although no comparable data is available for patients with cognitive compulsions, clinical observations and patients' reports seem to suggest the same functional relationship (Rachman, 1976a). Evidence that obsessions serve to increase anxiety derives from findings indicating that ruminative thoughts give rise to greater heart rate elevation and deflection of skin conductance than neutral thoughts (Boulougouris, Rabavilas, & Stefanis, 1977; Rabavilas & Boulougouris, 1974). In addition, touching a contaminated object (obsession) has been found to result in increases in heart rate and in subjective anxiety (Hodgson & Rachman, 1972) as well as in measures of skin conductance* (Hornsveld, Kraaimaat, & van Dam-Baggen, 1979).

The limitations of the two-stage theory have been noted by several authors (e.g., Carr, 1974; Rachman, 1976c; Teasdale, 1974). One of the difficulties with this model lies in its prediction that a fear reaction that is no longer paired with the unconditioned stimulus will eventually extinguish, resulting in the termination of avoidance responses. However, this hypothesis has not been borne out by laboratory or clinical observations. Rather, avoidance behavior tends to persist, irrespective of the intensity of the fear associated with it. Ad-

---

*Heart rate and measures of skin conductance have been shown to vary with other indications of anxiety (Mathews, 1971; Mathews & Shaw, 1973) and are thus considered to reflect the level of evoked discomfort.

ditionally, as the compulsions become more complex, the difficulty of successfully performing them increases, and the rituals themselves acquire aversive properties. Yet the strength of these repetitive behaviors does not seem to diminish, despite their increasingly unpleasant character.

It can be justifiably argued that the two-stage theory does not adequately explain either the acquisition of obsessions or the maintenance of all escape and avoidance behaviors (Foa & Steketee, 1979). Despite these shortcomings, the model does appear to provide a satisfactory explanation of the maintenance of compulsions through their anxiety-reducing properties.

Cognitive-Behavior Theory

In contrast to traditional behavioral approaches, cognitive models tend to emphasize the role of mediational variables in the pathogenesis of obsessive-compulsive disorders. Central to this formulation is the belief that symptoms are the by-product of unrealistic appraisals of threat and faulty evaluations of one's ability to cope adequately with such threat. This model, first proposed by Carr (1971, 1974) and later refined by McFall and Wollersheim (1979), suggests that unrealistic subjective estimates of danger stem from a variety of erroneous beliefs and irrational patterns of thinking. In obsessive-compulsives, these beliefs include the following: (a) the idea that one must be perfectly competent, adequate, and achieving in all endeavors in order to be worthwhile; (b) the belief that punishment should follow any failure to live up to perfectionistic ideals; (c) that obsessive ruminating or magical rituals can prevent the occurrence of catastrophies; and (d) that certain thoughts and feelings can lead to disastrous consequences and should be punished (McFall & Wollersheim,

1979). According to this model, the mistaken beliefs lead to erroneous perceptions of threat, which in turn lead to anxiety. This dysfunctional process is compounded by the obsessive-compulsive's tendency to devalue his or her ability to deal adequately with the subjective appraisals of danger. These secondary distortions, in turn, lead to feelings of uncertainty, discomfort, and helplessness, which are reduced through magical rituals and obsessions. Presumably, these symptoms are viewed by the patient as the only available alternative for dealing with perceived threat because the obsessive-compulsive feels that he or she lacks other, more appropriate coping resources.

Foa and Kozak (in press) conceptualized *anxiety disorders* as specific impairments in affective memory networks. They adopted Lang's (1979) bioinformational theory that states that fear exists as an information network (prototype) in memory that includes information about feared stimuli, fear responses, and their meanings. Neurotic fears, Foa and Kozak proposed, differ structurally from normal fears. The former are characterized by the presence of erroneous estimates of threat, unusually high negative valence for the threatening event, and excessive response elements (e.g., physiological, avoidance, etc.), and they are resistant to modification. This persistence may reflect failure to access the fear network, either because of active avoidance or because the content of the fear network precludes spontaneous encounters with situations that evoke anxiety in everyday life. Additionally, anxiety may persist because of some impairment in the mechanism of change. Cognitive defenses, high arousal, faulty premises, and erroneous rules of inference might hinder the processing of information necessary for changing the fear structure.

These authors suggest that no one form of fear structure is common to obsessive-compulsives. Typically, however, they base their beliefs about danger on the *absence* of disconfirming evidence; they fail to assume general safety from specific experiences of exposure to feared situations in which no harm occurred. Consequently, although rituals are performed to reduce the likelihood of harm, they can never really provide safety, and therefore they must be repeated.

CLASSIFICATION

Traditional attempts to categorize obsessive-compulsive symptomatology were phenomenological in nature, usually focusing on the specific ritualistic behaviors or on the content of the ruminative material. This is quite clear in the division of obsessive-compulsive patients into "washers," "checkers," "orderers," and the like. Although many patients manifest more than one type of ritualistic behavior, in most cases one specific type prevails. Washing/cleaning and checking rituals are the most common compulsions encountered (Stern & Cobb, 1978). "Repeaters" are a subgroup of checkers who repeat an action, usually a specified "magical" number of times in order to prevent a particular disaster from occurring. These individuals differ from other checkers in that their rituals are not related to feared consequences in a direct, rational way. A third group consists of patients who manifest ordering rituals in which certain objects must be precisely arranged in order to achieve a satisfying state of symmetry or balance. Disturbance of this order provokes extreme discomfort. A rarer category of "obsessional slowness" has been suggested by Rachman and Hodgson (1980). These patients do not appear to have distinct obsessions followed by ritualistic behavior designed to reduce anxiety. Rather, they carry out their everyday activities, particularly toileting, with meticulous care and many hours of effort. Other authors have attempted to provide a classification based on the form of obsessions (e.g., Akhtar, Wig, Verma, Pershad, & Verma, 1975; Capstick & Seldrup, 1973; Dowson, 1977).

A shortcoming inherent in all traditional classifications is that they fail to bear on treatment strategies. To avoid the infertility of mere intellectual exercise, nosology must be related to etiology and/or treatment. We shall propose a classification that rests on the class of cues that evokes anxiety and the type of activity (cognitive or overt) that reduces it. In so doing, we will be able to relate typology to treatment.

All obsessive-compulsives complain of the presence of intrusive thoughts, images, or impulses. These thoughts may be triggered by an external event, such as touching a contaminated object or locking a door, or they may arise without apparent external cues. A further categorization can be made with respect to the presence or absence of fears of disastrous consequences. For instance, the thought *Did I lock the door properly?* may be associated with the fear of a rapist invading one's home; the spontaneous image of Jesus' penis may give rise to a fear of going to hell. On the other hand, the intrusive thought *Is my hand contaminated?* may elicit discomfort in the absence of any disturbing consequences.

Thus, obsessions can be divided into several different kinds: (a) presence of intrusive cognitive material, external cues, and fears of disasters; (b) presence of intrusive material and external cues (in the absence of disasters); and (c) presence of intrusive material and fear of disasters (in the absence of external cues). An additional kind of intrusive cognitive material with neither external cues nor fear of disasters is theoretically possible, but we have not observed patients with such obsessions, nor have we come across reports of them in the literature. Rachman's (1976b) division of compulsions into "restorative" and "preventative" can provide an explanation for the absence of this pattern. It is difficult to imagine that a repetitive thought without either the urge to restore a state of relative calm or to prevent a future disaster would evoke anxiety sufficient to constitute an obsession. Thus, fears of disasters and/or associated external cues seem to be prerequisites for an intrusive, repetitious cognition to exist.

How can rituals be classified? Because our present conceptualization posits that all rituals are anxiety reducing, the type of ritual (e.g., washing, checking) becomes irrelevant because it does not lead to differential treatment. A more useful approach is to categorize compulsions on the basis of their mode (e.g., cognitive or behavioral). Although these two classes do not differ in their funtional relationship to anxiety, they do carry different treatment implications that will be discussed later.

The combination of the preceding classifications of obsessions and compulsions yields eight types of obsessive-compulsives; these are shown in Figure 1. As we have discussed, only six types have been observed. It should be stressed that these types are not mutually exclusive. A patient may experience obsessions of several different types. Similarly, a given obsession may give rise to both covert and overt rituals. As seen in Figure 1, the second, fourth, and sixth types are all distinguished by the absence of overt rituals. Patients manifesting this pattern have been labeled as *obsessional*; they may vary, however, with respect to whether or not their obsessions include external cues and/or anticipated disasters. Type 1, overt compulsions triggered by external cues and by fears of future disasters, is found in nearly all patients with checking rituals and in many of those with washing and cleaning rituals. The third type, obsessions triggered by external cues without feared consequences, is prevalent in patients

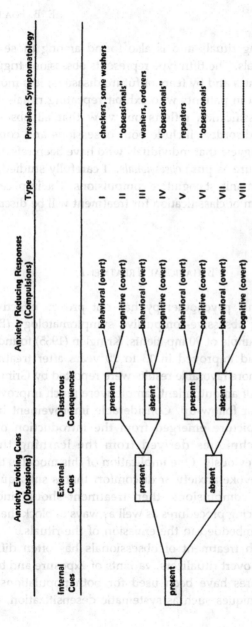

FIGURE 1. Typology of obsessive-compulsive manifestations.

Anxiety Evoking Cues (Obsessions)

Internal Cues	External Cues	Disastrous Consequences	Anxiety Reducing Responses (Compulsions)	Type	Prevalent Symptomatology
present	present	present	behavioral (overt)	I	checkers, some washers
			cognitive (covert)	II	"obsessionals"
		absent	behavioral (overt)	III	washers, orderers
			cognitive (covert)	IV	"obsessionals"
	absent	present	behavioral (overt)	V	repeaters
			cognitive (covert)	VI	"obsessionals"
		absent	behavioral (overt)	VII	
			cognitive (covert)	VIII	

with ordering rituals and is also found among those with washing rituals. The fifth type represents obsessions triggered by internal cues and by fears of future disasters; it is most often observed in patients who exhibit repeating rituals.

This classification reflects our view that all obsessive-compulsive disorders include both obsessions and compulsions. We suggest that individuals who have been referred to in the literature as pure *obsessionals*, if carefully studied, will be found to manifest cognitive compulsions. The implications of this system of classification for treatment will be discussed later.

BEHAVIORAL TREATMENT

Traditional psychotherapy has not proven effective in ameliorating obsessive-compulsive symptomatology (Black, 1974). In a sample of 90 inpatients, Kringlen (1965) found that only 20% had improved in 13 to 20 years after treatment. Somewhat more favorable results were reported by Grimshaw (1965); 40% of an outpatient sample were much improved at a 1-to 14-year follow-up. Considerable improvement in the prognostic picture emerged from the introduction of behavioral techniques derived from the learning theory described previously. One implication of this model is that if obsessions evoke anxiety or discomfort that is subsequently reduced by compulsions, then treatment should include anxiety-reducing procedures as well as ways to block the reinforcement embedded in the emission of the rituals.

Although treatment of obsessionals has often differed from that of overt ritualizers, variants of exposure and blocking procedures have been used for both populations. Exposure techniques such as systematic desensitization, paradoxical intention, flooding, and satiation consist of deliberately confronting the patient with anxiety-evoking material, either *in vivo* or in imagination. Blocking, on the other hand, cuts short the patient's ruminations or ritualistic behaviors via such procedures as response prevention, thought stopping, aversion, and distraction. We will first review the use of exposure procedures in the treatment of obsessive-compulsive ritualizers and in treatment of obsessionals. Blocking techniques will be discussed next, followed by an overview of the literature on the effects of *in vivo* exposure combined with response prevention—the current treatment of choice for ritualizers.

Exposure Procedures

The implementation of procedures directed at the anxiety associated with obsessions is based on the rationale that once the obsessional cues cease to evoke anxiety, compulsive behavior will extinguish because it will no longer be reinforced by its anxiety-reducing properties. To this end, *systematic desensitization* (Wolpe, 1958) has often been employed. This procedure consists of the induction of a relaxed state and the concomitant presentation of anxiety-evoking items arranged in a hierarchical order. It is hypothesized that the pairing of relaxation with the disturbing stimuli will eventually result in deconditioning of the associated anxiety. No direct effort to treat the ritualistic behavior has usually been attempted when systematic desensitization was employed.

The largest series of patients treated with this technique was reported by Cooper, Gelder, and Marks (1965). Of 10 obsessive-compulsives, only 3 improved; a control group treated with supportive psychotherapy and drugs showed greater gains. The results of single-case reports are less bleak but still ambiguous (e.g., Furst & Cooper, 1970; Haslam, 1965; Marks, Crowe, Drewe, Young, & Dewhurst, 1969; Rackensberger & Feinberg, 1972; Scrignar, 1974; Tanner, 1971; Wickramasekera, 1970; Wolpe, 1964; Worsley, 1970). In reviewing 21 cases treated by 5 to 100 sessions of systematic desensitization, Beech and Vaughn (1978) reported that 4 out of 10 patients treated with imaginal desensitization were improved, in contrast to 7 of the 11 who received this procedure *in vivo*. Although this difference is not striking, the latter technique seems to fare better.

Walton and Mather (1963) examined the differential effects of systematic desensitization on chronic versus recently acquired symptoms. The factors responsible for the elicitation and maintenance of compulsive behavior, they felt, varied with symptom duration. Recently acquired symptoms were presumed to be elicited by conditioned anxiety, whereas longstanding symptoms were hypothesized to be functionally autonomous and independent of anxiety. In accordance with this hypothesis, these authors predicted that only patients whose symptoms were of recent onset would benefit from systematic desensitization. As expected, compulsions were extinguished in two of three patients with recently acquired symptoms. Conversely, for two of the three patients with chronic symptoms, desensitization reduced anxiety, but the compulsions remained unchanged. Overall, then, of their six patients, half were improved with desensitization. It is interesting to note that Marks *et al.* (1969) also found that elimination of anxiety had no effect on avoidance behavior and rituals. The practical implications of these findings are clear; their theoretical implications will be discussed later when mechanisms operating during behavioral treatment are considered.

Desensitization has also been employed in the treatment of obsessionals who do not manifest overt rituals. Bevan (1960) treated a patient who ruminated about war and illness by combining 6 weeks of desensitization *in vivo* (reading anxiety-provoking material) with chlorpromazine. Some reduction in the treated obsessions was evident, but new ones emerged. Better results were reported by Agras, Leitenberg, Barlow, Curtis, Edwards, and Wright (1971) who utilized systematic desensitization with and without relaxation in treating patients who ruminated about harming others. Both procedures markedly reduced the frequency of obsessions, improvement being greater with the addition of relaxation.

Overall, the reported effectiveness of systematic desensitization for treatment of both ritualizers and obsessionals leaves much to be desired. Nevertheless, there is some justification for its use with patients with recent onset of symptoms; *in vivo* administration seems to optimize the outcome.

Several other procedures utilizing prolonged exposure have been employed with ritualizers. Noonan (1971) used a procedure he labeled *induced anxiety*. Although conceptualized within a traditional insight framework, this procedure resembled implosive therapy (Stampfl & Levis, 1967). The patient was instructed to experience intense anxiety and to describe the images that arose spontaneously. After seven sessions he was symptom free. A related approach, *paradoxical intention*, has also been employed with obsessive-compulsives (Frankl, 1960). This procedure typically involves deliberate attempts to increase the frequency or intensity of problematic thoughts or behaviors. An obsessive-compulsive individual might be asked to imagine in an exaggerated fashion that feared consequences ensuing from a failure to perform a ritual had actually occurred. A patient with checking rituals who feared making mistakes might be asked to think that he was the "greatest mistake maker in the world." This procedure seems to closely resemble implosion or flooding in imagination; the difference is that in paradoxical intention the patient is usually asked to carry out the procedure on his or her own, whereas in implosion or flooding the stimulus input for the images is provided by the therapist. Additionally, deliberate attempts to evoke humor are included in the former but not in the latter. Utilizing paradoxical intention with 6 obsessive-compulsives, Gertz (1966) reported that 4 patients recovered, and 2 improved. Paradoxical intention has also been employed with obsessionals who did not exhibit overt rituals. Solyom, Garza-Perez, Ledwidge, and Solyom (1972) treated 10 such patients with this technique and reported that 5 had markedly improved, 3 remained unchanged, and 2 failed to follow instructions.

Other variations of *prolonged exposure* have also been reported. McCarthy (1972) treated a patient with persistent worries about sexual attractiveness by exposing him to imagined scenes involving sexual failure. A 6-month follow-up revealed that he was no longer concerned with those fears. Concentrated exposure to verbalization of ruminations was employed by Broadhurst (1976) in treating obsessions about menstrual blood. The procedure involved alternating 5-or 10-minute exposure periods with rest periods of 1 to 3 minutes. Mild improvement was achieved at posttreatment with further improvement evident at a 4-year follow-up.

Two studies compared the effects of exposure with that of thought stopping, a blocking procedure that will be discussed in the next section. In the first study conducted by Emmelkamp and Kwee (1977), only one of the three patients who received five 60-minute exposure sessions as the first treatment evidenced improvement. In the second investigation, Stern (1978) compared the efficacy of yet another exposrue technique, *satiation*, with thought stopping. Seven patients with obsessive ruminations were given four sessions of satiation followed by four sessions of thought stopping. A 1-month interval separated the two treatments. Each satiation session lasted 1 hour and consisted of having the patient verbalize his or her rumination in the presence of the therapist who encouraged him or her in this regard by using verbal prompts. Daily practice of writing thoughts repeatedly was assigned, and patients were further instructed to expose themselves to external cues that elicited the obsession. The results of this study were disappointing; only two of the seven patients improved with satiation.

Exposure combined with *aversion relief* was employed by Solyom and his colleagues. Four patients suffering from ruminations, doubting, and horrific temptations were treated by the following procedure. A previously taped narrative of the obsessional thought sequence was played for the patient and periodically interrupted by a 20-second silences that were followed by a mild electric shock. When the shock was terminated by the patient, the taped obsessional material resumed. In effect, relief from shock (negative reinforcement) was associated with the anxiety-arousing stimuli. All four patients were improved and recovered at follow-up (Solyom, Zamanzadeh, Ledwidge, & Kenny, 1971). In a later study, the same technique was successfully applied to treat sexual and aggressive ruminations (Solyom & Kingstone, 1973). The authors viewed this aversion-relief procedure as a form of reciprocal inhibition rather than negative reinforcement. They posited that because horrific temptations are anxiety-augmenting stimuli, they would be most affected by this procedure, whereas ruminations might be more successfully treated with other behavioral techniques.

Although exposure procedures have usually been directed at obsessions, Rabavilas, Boulougouris, and Stefanis (1977) employed such a technique to treat overt rituals. Four patients with checking rituals were requested to prolong the time spent ritualizing beyond their urge to do so. Although none of the patients actually followed the instructions, all showed marked improvement at follow-up; their rituals decreased by two-thirds. The mechanism by which these instructions succeeded is unclear because no actual overexposure occurred. However, the results are sufficiently intriguing to warrant replication.

In summary, variations of prolonged exposure do not seem to affect ritualistic behavior, nor does it appear to improve obsessions. Positive results have been obtained with the aversion-relief procedure employed by Solyom and his associates. However, this technique has been employed in one center only and requires replication.

Blocking Procedures

If compulsions are maintained because they are effective in decreasing discomfort, they should extinguish if they become associated with an increase rather than a decrease in discomfort. Lazarus (1958) reported a successful outcome by pairing anxiety induction with imaginal scenes involving emission of checking rituals. Use of the *aversion-relief* paradigm was reported by both Marks *et al.* (1969) and Rubin and Merbaum (1971). In these treatments electrical shock was made contingent on emission of rituals and was terminated upon contact with the "contaminated" object. Thus, patients experienced discomfort when performing the ritual and relief when touching the disturbing object. This procedure, then, constituted a reversal of the usual obsessive-compulsive contingencies. Some improvement was evidenced in patients treated by this technique, although their compulsions were not entirely eliminated.

The effects of *aversion procedures* with no relief were studied by Kenny, Mowbray, and Lalani (1978). Obsessions and compulsions were divided into component steps that were then imagined by the patient. Electrical shocks accompanied each of the imagined scenes. Improvement was noted in three of the five patients treated by this method. A self-administered aversion treatment of compulsive handwashing was successfully executed by LeBoeuf (1974). Yet another variant of aversion therapy, covert sensitization, was employed with a patient who had neatness and ordering rituals (Wisocki, 1970). Fantasized repulsive consequences were made contingent upon imagining ritualistic behavior. Covert reinforcement followed imagine absinence from ritualistic behavior and the performance of incompatible responses. A successful outcome was reported.

In summary, techniques aimed at blocking the ritualistic behavior by the use of aversion have generally yielded good results. However, extinguishing motor responses associated with negative affect may result in relapse. Indeed, Walton (1960) reported a relapse in cases in which only the motor responses were treated. As we shall see later, blocking of ritualistic behavior in the absence of procedures directed at anxiety reduction is minimally effective in the long run.

Blocking procedures have frequently been employed with obsessionals in an attempt to reduce disturbing cognitive material. McGuire and Vallance (1964) delivered shock to a patient upon deliberate elicitation of ruminative material relating to distrust of his wife. Three sessions of treatment followed by 10 days of home practice (self-delivery of shock) were quite effective in controlling these obsessions. In yet another study, two female obsessionals, both of whom reported sexual and aggressive urges, were treated with shock following the verbal expression of obsessional material (Kenny, Solyom, & Solyom, 1973). One patient treated in seven sessions remained improved after 6 months; the other improved after 23 sessions but relapsed 3 months later. A variant of aversive therapy was employed by Kenny, Mowbray, and Lalani (1978) who administered shock to patients following their signal of a clear obsessional thought. Six patients were treated for an average of 35 sessions; four rated themselves as greatly improved, one rated himself as moderately improved, whereas another failed to benefit. Single-case studies by Bass (1973) and Mahoney (1971) have also reported success in controlling obsessions by using an aversion method that involved instructing patients to snap a rubber band against their wrist whenever obsessional thoughts occurred.

Another major technique used in the blocking of obsessions is *thought stopping*. Stern (1970) utilized this procedure to treat a patient who ruminated about performing actions correctly. Obsessions were ordered from least to most disturbing and were successfully treated by instructing the patient to shout "'stop" upon the evocation of an intrusive rumination. Yamagami (1971) also achieved good results by applying a procedure that involved the sequential application of thought stopping alone, thought stopping combined with incompatible responses, and aversion therapy. However, the effect of thought stopping is difficult to interpret because the author employed thought stopping alone for only a short period of time. In retrospect, it is unclear why this procedure was discontinued in favor of the remaining variations, given its success in reducing the obsessions.

Two case studies reported by Leger (1978) provide further support for the use of thought stopping to control obsessions. Both cases involved treating obsessive ideation through a combination of thought stopping and relaxation. The positive results obtained for both patients were sustained at follow-up. Gullick and Blanchard (1973) used thought stopping in conjunction with other techniques to treat a case involving religious obsessions. Treatment included psychotherapy, thought stopping, attribution therapy, and assertiveness training. Although a successful outcome was reported, thought stopping itself seemed to have had little effect.

The preceding case studies present an optimistic outlook of the usefulness of thought stopping in reducing ruminations, but the picture becomes more bleak when the outcome of controlled studies is examined. In comparing relaxation instructions alone with a combination of relaxation and thought stopping, Stern, Lipsedge, and Marks (1975) found that only 4 of 11 patients treated with thought stopping improved. In an attempt to explain these poor results, the authors suggested that their use of a tape recorder might have diminished the effectiveness of treatment because presentation of scenes via tape recordings were found less effective than presentation by a therapist in person (Marks, 1972). Therefore, Stern (1978) replicated this study with four obsessionals using a therapist in person. The results were even more disappointing: Only one improved slightly with this technique. In an additional sample of 7 patients, thought stopping with assigned daily home practice resulted in slight improvement for only two patients. Similarly, Emmelkamp and Kwee (1977) found that only one of two patients receiving thought stopping as a first treatment showed gains.

In summary, treatment by variants of thought stopping produced positive results in four of five case studies, but only one-third of the patients in multiple-case reports and controlled studies has benefited from this procedure. Because this difference is probably due to the practice of reporting successful single cases, the overall picture of the efficacy of thought stopping with obsessions can be viewed as discouraging. By contrast, aversion techniques have produced a more consistent and positive picture. Successful outcomes have been reported in five of six single-case studies and in five of six patients participating in a controlled study.

Comparisons between Exposure and Blocking Procedures

To date, only three studies have compared the effects of exposure and blocking treatments with obsessionals. Fifty-one volunteer subjects who scored high on anxiety and on obsessions were treated by five sessions of systematic desensitization, covert sensitization, or both (Kazarian & Evans, 1977). All three groups improved equally on measures of frequency of obsessions and were significantly better than two control groups at posttreatment and at a 5-week follow-up. The other two studies have utilized patient rather than analog populations. In a crossover design, Emmelkamp and Kwee (1977) examined the differential efficacy of five sessions of thought stopping and five sessions of prolonged imaginal exposure. Three of their five patients improved equally with either procedure, whereas the remaining two failed to improve regardless of the treatment applied. Results at variance with those of Emmelkamp and Kwee were reported by Stern (1978). Of seven patients who received exposure followed by thought stopping, only two improved. These poor results are disturbing because Stern employed an intense exposure procedure that included homework instructions to record obsessive thoughts and to seek out stimulus situations that evoked ruminations. Stern attempted to explain the poor outcome by suggesting that only some obsessions, in particular horrific ones, would be affected by prolonged exposure that allows for habituation of anxiety. However, Emmelkamp and Kwee's results do not support this proposition. Although four of their five patients suffered from horrific obsessions, they were affected *equally* by exposure and thought stopping.

New avenues for the treatment of obsessions have been suggested by two studies. Mills and Solyom (1974) used biofeedback in training five obsessionals to generate EEG alpha waves. During the alpha state that was experienced as a relaxed, day-dreaming or "blank mind" period, four of the five patients reported no obsessions; the remaining patient reported only a few. However, this effect did not generalize to ruminations occurring in the nonalpha state. The amount of alpha waves produced did not appear to be related to the success in reducing obsessions. In a second study, two female volunteers were trained to ruminate under hypnotic suggestion (Barone, Blum, & Porter, 1975). Four procedures for reducing obsessions were tested: a hypnotically induced blank mind state, a hypnotically induced "substitute thought" state (in which the subject would think about the classes she was taking), aversive white noise, and a control procedure in which the subject was allowed to think about anything she wanted to. The blank mind state was found to be the "most consistently effective technique for eliminating obsessions and preventing their spontaneous occurrence in a free thought period." The techniques employed in these two studies appear to be variants of blocking procedures (distraction?). Although their success was limited, they may provide a basis for the development of new procedures.

Summary

Included in the foregoing review are numerous reports on the effects of several variants of exposure and blocking procedures on ritualizers and obsessionals. Yet, the conclusions that can be derived from this body of research are at best equivocal. With few exceptions, these investigations have failed to distinguish between effects of the treatment on obsessions and on ritualistic behavior. Of further concern is the fact that much of the available information has been derived from single-case studies. Although these are useful for generating hypotheses and developing procedures, they cannot test a treatment's efficacy.

If information from case reports are not included, the rather sparse body of literature on the treatment of ritualizers with exposure procedures is disappointing. At best, only 50% of patients responded to desensitization. At first glance, paradoxical intention appears to have fared better, but the criteria for evaluating the outcome in the two available group studies is too ambiguous to allow firm conclusions about the efficacy of this technique. Exposure procedures employing aversion relief have also had limited success. Overall, fewer than half of the patients treated with this method evidenced gains at follow-up. It is apparent, then, that the exposure techniques described have had limited success in the treatment of obsessions and rituals. More positive results have been obtained with blocking procedures that have utilized faradic aversion. However, with only one multiple-case report available, the evidence in favor of this approach can hardly be regarded as conclusive. Moreover, the use of electrical shock in treatment has raised ethical concerns in recent years, and its use has been discouraged.

Intervention procedures employed with obsessionals have fared no better than those used to treat ritualizers. Again, discarding single-case reports, exposure techniques (aversion relief, paradoxical intention, satiation, and prolonged exposure) have produced an overall success rate of 42% improvement in obsessions. Blocking techniques (aversion with electrical shock or rubber band and thought stopping) yielded imrovement in 43% of patients. Thus, neither blocking nor exposure techniques have resulted in satisfactory outcome with obsessionals. Although this is the current state of the art in the treatment of obsessionals, the prognosis for obsessive-compulsive ritualizers has improved considerably. Data to this effect will be presented in the next section, and a possible explanation for the differential status of the two subgroups will be advanced.

TREATMENT BY EXPOSURE AND RESPONSE PREVENTION

Outcome Studies

The first attempt to treat ritualistic behavior by combining exposure with response prevention was reported by Meyer in 1966. In this program labeled *apotrepic therapy*, rituals were prevented for long periods while the patient was required to remain in circumstances that normally evoked anxiety and ritualistic activities. The successful outcome achieved in two cases with washing rituals was later replicated with additional ritualizers (Meyer & Levy, 1973; Meyer, Levy, & Schnurer, 1974). Of the 15 patients treated in this way by Meyer and his associates, 10 were rated much improved or symptom free; the remaining 5 were moderately improved. Only 2 of the patients relapsed after 5 to 6 years.

These remarkable results generated great interest in this treatment program. Numerous controlled and uncontrolled studies have resulted yielding information that bears on both the outcome of these procedures and the process involved. Much of the available information about the effects of exposure and response prevention with obsessive-compulsives comes from studies conducted on inpatients at the Maudsley Hospital in London in which procedural variants of exposure were investigated (Hodgson, Rachman, & Marks, 1972; Marks, Hodgson, & Rachman, 1975; Rachman, Hodgson, &

Marks, 1971; Rachman, Marks, & Hodgson, 1973). In all their investigations, the effects of treatment by exposure and response prevention were compared to a control condition of treatment by relaxation in order to ascertain that the improvement observed was not due merely to time spent in therapy. Fifteen daily sessions of variants of exposure *in vivo* were employed in conjunction with response prevention to treat 20 obsessive-compulsive inpatients. Eight patients were much improved, 7 were improved, and 5 failed to show change. By contrast, relaxation training had no effect. At a 2-year follow-up, 14 patients remained much improved, 1 was improved, and 5 were unchanged. Similar results with 10 washers were reported by Roper, Rachman, and Marks (1975). In this study, 5 patients received 15 daily sessions of treatment in which they observed the therapist modeling exposure to disturbing objects (passive modeling). The 5 control subjects were treated with 15 sessions of relaxation exercises. Both groups were then given 15 additional sessions of *in vivo* exposure (participant modeling) and response prevention. At the end of treatment, 3 patients were much improved, 5 were improved, whereas 2 remained unchanged. Similar results (4 much improved, 4 improved, 2 unchanged) emerged at follow-up.

An additional series of 13 patients were treated in the Maudsley by nurse therapists with an average of 14 sessions of exposure and response prevention (Marks, Bird, & Lindley, 1978). Significant improvement on measures of obsessive-compulsive symptoms was reported, but information about the number of successes and failures was not furnished. In a more recent study, the same procedures were employed with and without clomipramine in treating 40 obsessive-compulsives (Marks, Stern, Mawson, Cobb, & McDonald, 1980; Rachman, Cobb, Grey, McDonald, Mawson, Sartory, & Stern, 1979). Group means showed a significant reduction in anxiety and rituals, but again no attempt was made to document the number of successes.

In two studies by Boulougouris and his associates (Boulougouris & Bassiakos, 1973; Rabavilas, Boulougouris, & Stefanis, 1976), 15 patients were exposed to an average of 11 sessions of *in vivo* and imaginal exposure combined with response prevention instructions. Nine patients improved after treatment and maintained their gains at follow-up. Four additional patients received treatment and also improved, whereas 2 remained unchanged. A long-term follow-up of these patients (Boulougouris, 1977) yielded disappointing results: 6 of the 15 patients failed to exhibit treatment gains.

Three studies with outpatients were conducted in Holland by Emmelkamp and his colleagues. In the first study, 13 obsessive-compulsives were treated in their homes with fifteen 2-hour sessions of exposure and response prevention (Boersma, Den Hengst, Dekker, & Emmelkamp, 1976). Seven patients were symptom free, 3 showed some improvement, and 3 remained unchanged. Similar findings emerged at follow-up. In a comparison of therapist-aided versus self-controlled exposure, Emmelkamp and van Kraanen (1977) treated 13 patients with ten 2-hour sessions of exposure to anxiety-evoking cues. Posttreatment and follow-up data indicated an overall significant reduction in anxiety and ritualistic behavior. However, 2 patients failed to benefit from treatment and 8 required additional exposure sessions. Emmelkamp, van der Helm, van Zanten, and Plochy (1980) treated 15 obsessive-compulsive patients with 10 sessions of *in vivo* exposure and response prevention. Improvement was found at posttreatment and at a 1-and 6-month follow-up, although only group means were reported; the gains were comparable to those obtained in the Maudsley studies. Slight relapse was evident at the 1-month follow-up, and patients were given an average of 15 additional treatment sessions. In discussing these results, the authors suggested that 10 sessions of exposure and response prevention might not adequately protect patients against future relapse.

More detailed information about the effects of exposure and response prevention on obsessive-compulsive symptomatology was provided by Foa and Goldstein (1978). In this study, continuous exposure and complete response prevention was implemented with 21 ritualizers. All patients received 10 daily 2-hour sessions of imaginal and *in vivo* exposure and were supervised in response prevention. Treatment was conducted on an outpatient basis for 14 patients; the remaining 7 were treated as inpatients. After treatment, 18 of the 21 patients were symptom free on measures of rituals, 2 had improved, and 1 remained unchanged. At follow-up, 3 relapsed to various degrees. With regard to obsessions, 12 patients were asymptomatic after treatment; 8 were mildly to moderately symptomatic; and 1 failed to change. At follow-up, 2 patients relapsed.

In a subsequent study, Foa, Steketee, Turner, and Fischer (1980) attempted to investigate the effects of adding imaginal exposure to disastrous consequences to exposure *in vivo* to external cues. Seven patients with checking rituals from the Foa and Goldstein study (1978) were compared with 8 checkers treated with 10 daily 2-hour sessions of exposure and response prevention. At posttreatment, the overall mean improvement for the 15 patients treated was comparable to that found in the earlier study and in other research centers. At a 9-month follow-up, 4 of the 8 who had received exposure *in vivo* relapsed to various degrees, whereas those who had been given *both* imaginal and *in vivo* exposure maintained their gains.

In the foregoing studies, improvement was assessed on

9-point Likert-like scales of obsessive-compulsive symptoms; these scales were first developed at the Maudsley for phobic complaints and were later adapted for obsessive-compulsive disorders. The findings derived from the use of these measures were corroborated by Foa, Steketee, and Milby (1980) who used daily self-monitoring of rituals and subjective anxiety during controlled confrontation with the most feared contaminant as measures of outcome. Eight patients with washing rituals were treated by 20 sessions of exposure alone or response prevention alone followed by the combination of the two procedures; four were outpatients, and four were inpatients. By the end of treatment, the mean washing time for the two groups had decreased from 69 minutes to 15.5 minutes. The exposure test indicated that mean anxiety levels had decreased from 90 SUDs (subjective units of discomfort) before treatment to 16 SUDs after treatment. Five patients were much improved, and three were moderately improved; none failed. At a 2-year follow-up some relapse was evident in two patients who had improved moderately, whereas the five who were much improved retained their gains; the remaining patient could not be located.

Foa and her colleagues analyzed data collected from 50 patients who participated in various experiments in which treatment by exposure and response prevention was applied (Foa, Grayson, Steketee, Doppelt, Turner, & Latimer, 1983b). To obtain a measure of improvement, assessor's ratings of obsessions and compulsions on 9-point Likert-like scales were converted into percentage change from pretreatment baseline scores. These scores were averaged, and comparisons were made between pretreatment, posttreatment, and follow-up evaluations. On the basis of their percentage change score, partients were divided into three groups: those who exhibited treatment gains of 70% or more were categorized as *much im-*

proved; those who evidenced treatment gains of 31% to 69% were classified as *improved*; and *failures* were patients with improvement of 30% or less. Immediately after treatment, 29 out of 50 patients (58%) were much improved, 19 (38%) were improved, and 2 (4%) failed. At follow-up, ranging from 3 months to 3 years with a mean of 1 year, 27 of 46 patients (59%) were much improved, 8 (17%) were improved, and 11 (24%) failed to benefit from treatment. Those who were much improved tended to retain their gains, and those who failed at posttreatment did not improve at follow-up. Partial gains immediately after treatment were generally unstable and often resulted in relapse.

Further support for the effectiveness of exposure and response prevention comes from a study by Julien, Riviere, and Note (1980). Their results were congruent with those found in other centers: Two of their 20 patients dropped out of treatment; 12 were much improved; 5 were moderately improved; and 1 remained unchanged. Follow-up assessments conducted 6 months to 3 years after treatment indicated some relapse. Excellent results were reported by Catts and McConaghy (1975) with 6 obsessive-compulsives: After treatment 4 patients were rated as improved on ritualistic behavior; 1 was judged much improved; 1 became asymptomatic. Further improvement in both rituals and obsessions was noted at follow-up evaluations 9 to 24 months later. The same positive picture emerges from various case studies (e.g., Farkas & Beck, 1981; Haynes, 1978; Lipper & Feigenbaum 1976; Meyer, Robertson, & Tatlow, 1975; Rainey, 1972). Three series of carefully designed single-case studies (Mills, Agras, Barlow, & Mills, 1973; Turner, Hersen, Bellack, & Wells, 1979; Turner, Hersen, Bellack, Andrasik, & Capparell, 1980) are of particular interest because behavioral observations of time spent ritualizing constituted their primary outcome measure. They provide further corroboration for the findings that have emerged from studies using global measures.

To date, over 200 obsessive-compulsive ritualizers have been treated with prolonged exposure and response prevention. In contrast to the information available for obsessionals (without over rituals), most of the data for ritualizers has been derived from group studies rather than single-case reports, adding confidence to the findings. The remarkable convergence of these studies that were conducted in many centers with numerous therapists further attests to the generalizability of the treatmeant effects. Table 1 summarizes the findings of the group studies of treatment by exposure and response prevention. According to this table, 51% of patients treated by this method were either symptom free or much improved at the end of treatment and 39% were moderately improved; only 10% failed to benefit from therapy. Although at follow-up the number of failures increased to 24%, the high efficacy of this treatment regimen is evident. It seems, then, that exposure and response prevention can indeed be considered the treatment of choice for obsessive-compulsive ritualizers.

We should note that treatment in most of these studies was conducted daily and often in a hospital setting. Can the intensity of the treatment account for its superior results? This does not seem to be the case. In each of the Maudsley studies, treatment by exposure and response prevention was compared with an equivalent amount of relaxation training. The latter method proved completely ineffective in ameliorating obsessive-compulsive symptomatology. Still, it is possible that extraneous variables such as expectancy may have played a role in the Maudsley studies because no measure of this factor was obtained. However, in a study examining the separate and combined effects of exposure and response prevention, Steketee, Foa, and Grayson (1982) controlled for

TABLE 1. Results of Studies
Using Variant of Exposure/Response Prevention Treatment

Study	Number of cases	Number of treatment sessions	Follow-up period	Outcome at posttreatment	Outcome at follow-up
Meyer, Levy & Schnurer (1974)	15	2 wks.–2 mos.	5–6 yr	20% no symptoms 47% much improved 33% improved	17% no symptoms 50% much improved 17% improved 17% relapsed
Marks, Hodgson & Rachman (1975)	20	15	2 yr	40% much improved 35% improved 25% no change	70% much improved 5% improved 25% no change
Roper, Rachman & Marks (1975)	10	15	6 mo	30% much improved 50% improved 20% no change	40% much improved 40% improved 20% no change
Marks, Stern, Mowson, Cobb, & McDonald (1980)	40	15 (for 20 pts.)			
Rachman, Cobb, Grey, McDonald, Mawson, Sartory, & Stern	30 for 20 pts.)				
Marks, Bird & Lindley (1978)	13	14 (mean)	6 mo	Statistically significant improvement in group means	
Boulougouris & Bassiakos (1973)	3	23 (mean)	9 mo	All improved to various degrees	

Study	N	Follow-up		
Rabavilas, Boulougouris, & Stefanis (1976)	12	6 mo (mean)	50% improved 33% slightly improved 17% no change	50% improved 33% moderately improved 17% no change
Boulougouris (1977)	15 (same patients as in above two studies)	2.8 yr	87% improved	60% improved
Boersma, Den Hengst, Dekker & Emmelkamp (1976)	13	3 mo		54% no symptoms 23% improved 23% no change
Emmelkamp & van Kraanen (1977)	13	3.5 mo	Statistically significant improvement in group means	
Emmelkamp, van der Helm, van Zanten, & Plochy (1980)	15	6 mo	Statistically significant improvement in group means	
Foa & Goldstein (1978)	10 (18 pts.) 15 (3 pts.)	3 yr	Rituals Obsessions 85% no symptoms 57% 10% much improved 10% —improved 28%	Rituals Obsessions 79% no symptoms 63% —much improved 5% 10% improved 16% 11% no change 16%
Foa, Steketee, Turner & Fischer (1980)	15 (includes 7 from Foa & Goldstein, 1978)	9 mo	Statistically significant improvement in group means	

Continued

TABLE 1. *Continued*

Study	Number of cases	Number of treatment sessions	Follow-up period	Outcome at posttreatment		Outcome at follow-up	
Foa, Steketee & Milby (1980)	8	20	0	64% much improved 36% moderately improved		57% much improved 14% moderately improved 29% slightly improved	
Foa, Grayson, Steketee, Doppelt, Turner, & Latimer (1983b)	50 (includes 37 pts from preceding 3 studies	10-20	1 yr (range 3 mo-3yr)	58% much improved 38% improved 4% failed		59% much improved 17% much improved 24% much improved	
Catts & McConaghy (1975)	6	20	9 mo to 2 yr	Rituals 17% no symptoms 17% much improved 66% improved	Anxiety — 50% 33%	Rituals 50% no symptoms 50% much improved —improved	Anxiety 33% 50% 17%
Julien, Riviere & Note (1980)	18	20 mean	1 yr (mean) (range 6 mo–3 yr)	67% much improved 28% improved 5% no change		39% much improved 28% improved 33% no change	

expectancy as well as the frequency and duration of treatment. Comparisons were made between treatments that combined exposure with response prevention and those that employed each procedure alone. Expectancy was equivalent across groups and therefore could not account for the superior results obtained by the combined procedure.

Variants of Exposure and Response Prevention

Meyer's apotrepic therapy consisted of two basic components: exposure to discomfort-evoking stimuli and prevention of ritualistic responses. What do we know about the ways in which these two procedures should be administered?

The Form of Exposure: Imaginal versus In Vivo. Early reports on the effect of the modality of the exposure with obsessive-compulsive patients were conflicting. Stampfl (1967) successfully treated an obsessive compulsive patient by imaginally exposing him to his most feared situation. Yet, Rachman, Hodgson, and Marzillier (1970) concluded that implosion had no therapeutic effect on washing rituals, whereas exposure *in vivo* combined with modeling produced good results.

More recently, Rabavilas *et al.* (1976) employed a Latin square design to examine the impact of different forms of exposure on obsessive-compulsive symptoms. Long and short periods of imaginal and *in vivo* exposure were administered to 12 patients; because each patient received all four treatments, the order of presentation was controlled. *In vivo* exposure proved significantly more effective in reducing obsessive-compulsive symptoms than exposure in fantasy. These results were consistent with those found for agoraphobics (Emmelkamp, 1974; Emmelkamp & Wessels, 1975; Everaerd, Rijken, & Emmelkamp, 1973; Stern & Marks, 1973). The only study in which imaginal exposure proved to be as effective as actual exposure was reported by Mathews, Johnston, Lancashire, Munby, Shaw, and Gelder (1976). However, this equivalence was attributed to the *in vivo* practice between sessions for all patients.

Most of the studies have focused on the modality rather than on the content of the exposure and its relevance to the patient's symptomatology. When exposure in fantasy includes only tangible cues, it merely shadows exposure to *in vivo* situations. It is therefore not surprising that the latter technique is often more effective. However, for many neurotic patients, anxiety is generated by both tangible environmental cues and thoughts of possible disasters following exposure to such cues (e.g., death, disease, house burning down, etc.). If it is important to match the content of the exposure to the patient's internal fear model as Lang (1977) has suggested, then checkers whose rituals center around responsibility for potential catastrophes should improve more when imaginal exposure to these stimuli is added to *in vivo* exposure to external tangible stimuli. To test this hypothesis, Foa, Steketee, Turner, and Fischer (1980) assigned 15 patients with checking rituals and fears of disastrous consequences to one of the following two conditions: imaginal exposure, *in vivo* exposure, and response prevention (Group 1); and exposure *in vivo* only combined with response prevention (Group 2). The results are depicted in Figures 2 and 3.

Contrary to their hypothesis, both groups improved considerably after treatment but did not differ significantly. However, follow-up data (mean of 11 months) indicated that the members of the group that received imaginal and *in vivo* exposure retained their gains more than did those in the group receiving exposure *in vivo* alone. These findings have recently been replicated with a larger number of patients, both washers and checkers (Doppelt, 1981). Thus, exposure to disastrous consequence seems to have affected variables important to the maintenance of gains rather than those responsible for immediate fear reduction. At present, then, imaginal exposure seems to be a valuable addition to *in vivo* exposure for patients with fears of disastrous consequences.

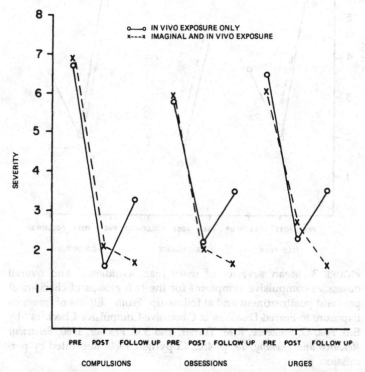

FIGURE 2. Mean severity of compulsions, obsessions, and urges for the two groups of checkers at pre- and posttreatment and at follow-up. From "Effects of Imaginal Exposure to Feared Disasters in Obsessive-Compulsive Checkers" by E.B. Foa, G. Steketee, R.M. Turner, and S.C. Fischer, 1980, *Behaviour Research and Therapy, 18,* p. 452. Copyright 1980. Reprinted by permission.

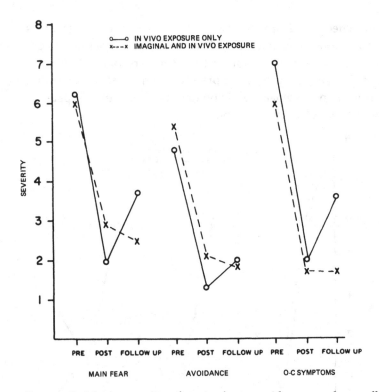

FIGURE 3. Mean severity of main fear, avoidance, and overall obsessive-compulsive symptoms for the two groups of checkers at pre- and posttreatment and at follow-up. From "Effects of Imaginal Exposure to Feared Disasters in Obsessive-Compulsive Checkers" by E.B. Foa, G. Steketee, R.M. Turner, and S.C. Fischer, 1980, *Behaviour Research and Therapy, 18,* p. 452. Copyright 1980. Reprinted by permission.

Duration of Exposure. Studies with both animals and volunteer subjects suggest that prolonged exposure to fear-provoking stimuli is superior to brief exposure. In treating agoraphobic patients, Stern and Marks (1973) found that 2 hours of continuous exposure yielded better outcome than 4 half-hour periods separated by rest periods of a half-hour each. These results were replicated with obsessive-compulsives by Rabavilas *et al.* (1976) who examined the differential effects of long versus short exposure in fantasy and *in vivo*. Eighty minutes of continuous *in vivo* exposure proved superior to eight 10-minute segments of exposure *in vivo*. However, when exposure was imaginal, the length of time did not produce a different outcome.

Experiments with animals have demonstrated that extinction does occur with brief exposure periods when the interval between trials is short (Mackintosh, 1974). Perhaps, then, the 10- and 30-minute exposure intervals employed in the preceding experiments were too lengthy and interfered with the process of extinction. Indeed, Shipley, Mock, and Levis (1971) found that with short intervals, extinction was related to the total amount of exposure rather than to the number of trials. With humans, a decrement in anxiety associated with obsessions was observed after repeated exposure of 2 minutes' duration separated by 1-minute intervals (Parkinson & Rachman, 1980). It seems, then, that the total amount of exposure time and the length of the interval between exposure trials influence treatment outcome.

Gradual versus Rapid Exposure. Desensitization procedures are based on the supposition that anxiety reduction is best achieved by gradual exposure to discomforting stimuli so that only low levels of fear are experienced. Proponents of implosion posit that the opposite must occur in that the experience of high levels of anxiety will promote its extinction. Studies examining habituation to neutral stimuli suggest that gradual exposure will result in faster and more complete response decrement than presentation of high-intensity stimuli. However, the speed of presentation of the most disturbing stimuli has not proved to be a salient variable in the treatment of obsessive-compulsives. Hodgson, *et al.* (1972) exposed patients gradually to discomfort-evoking situations after they watched the therapist model each step. Other patients were exposed immediately to the most feared situation, again after watching the therapist model exposure. Both groups were treated for 15 sessions. The two procedures were equally effective, although patients reported feeling more comfortable with the graduated approach. Boersma *et al.* (1976) obtained similar results. Only the patients rating "anxiety—main compulsion" yielded a significant difference in favor of gradual exposure. On the other hand, Foa and Kozak (in press) found a small but negative correlation between treatment outcome and the level of subjective anxiety reported by obsessive-compulsives during the initial presentation of their most feared stimulus. This might suggest that successful outcomes may best be facilitated by moderate levels of anxiety.

Exposure with and without Modeling. In an attempt to study the effect of modeling on exposure treatments, Roper *et al.* (1975) in a study described earlier, found that although some reduction of obsessive-compulsive symptomatology was obtained with passive modeling, participant modeling and response prevention yielded considerably better results. However, these findings are difficult to interpret because this study is confounded by the inclusion of response prevention instructions only with participant but not with passive modeling. In an earlier study, Rachman *et al.* (1973) compared flooding *in vivo* with and without modeling and found no differences between treatments. Similar results were obtained in a study by Boersma *el al.* (1977) who found that only the degree of avoidance related to secondary compulsions was affected by modeling. As noted by Marks *et al.* (1975), this does not imply that certain individuals cannot benefit from modeling. Some patients have reported that modeling by the therapist assisted them in overcoming their resistance and fear of exposure.

Therapist Role. Therapist qualities of warmth, genuineness, and empathy have long been recognized as important components of any psychotherapeutic intervention (e.g., Truax & Carkuff, 1967). Informal observations have led Marks *et al.* (1975) to suggest that exposure and response-prevention treatment "requires a good patient–therapist working relationship, and a sense of humor helps patients over difficult situations" (p. 360). Some of their patients also commented that they could contaminate themselves following the therapist's instructions but had been unable to do so previously when urged by their spouses.

A prospective study by Rabavilas, Boulougouris, and Perissaki (1979) confirmed these observations. In their study, phobic and obsessive-compulsive patients who had been treated by exposure *in vivo* were asked to rate their therapist on 16 variables related either to the therapist's attitude or to the way in which he or she conducted treatment. Patients who rated their therapist as respectful, understanding, interested, encouraging, challenging, and explicit improved more. On the other hand, gratification of dependency needs, permissiveness, and tolerance were negatively related to outcome.

Although the personal style of the therapist seems to be an important variable, his or her presence during exposure does not appear to have a significant impact on outcome. Emmelkamp and van Kraanen (1977) compared 10 sessions of self-controlled *in vivo* exposure with an equivalent number of sessions in which the therapist controlled the exposure. No differences in outcome were found on obsessive-compulsive symptomatology. However, the latter group required more treatment sessions at follow-up than did the former. The authors suggested that the self-controlled exposure group may have gained greater independence in handling their fears. Self-controlled exposure was also found to be as effective as therapist-controlled exposure with agoraphobics (Mathews, Gelder, & Johnston, 1981). But the therapist was involved in directing and supervising the patient. It is questionable whether the positive outcome would have occurred without such involvement. Thus, the findings of these studies do not suggest that the therapist is dispensible. Rather, they merely indicate that *in vivo* exposure may be implemented without his or her immediate presence.

Coupled with the evident potency of exposure in treating anxiety-based disorders, the failure to detect differences between variants of exposure may be due to a ceiling effect. The number of subjects per cell was quite small so that only powerful effects could have been detected. Thus, the results cannot be interpreted as evidence that variables such as therapist presence, rapidity of presentation, and so forth do not impact at all on treatment outcome, but they do not appear to be crucial. Additionally, response prevention was implemented simultaneously with deliberate exposure for obsessive-compulsives, and its effects may have further obscured differences among variants of exposure.

Response Prevention Variants. The other treatment component, blocking of ritualistic behavior, has been labeled *response prevention*, a term borrowed from the animal literature (Baum, 1970). Although differential effects of variants of exposure modalities have been systematically studied, relatively little attention has been directed at variants of response prevention. The apotrepic therapy described by Meyer *et al.* (1974) involved inpatient treatment and "continual supervision during the patient's waking hours by nurses who were instructed to prevent the patient from carrying out any rituals" (p. 246). When rituals consisted of repetitions of normal, necessary behaviors, some judgment was exercised as to how often and for how long the patient should engage in the particular behavior. After total suppression of symptoms was achieved in spite of the stress caused by exposure, supervision was gradually relaxed. Likewise, Turner and his colleagues (Turner *et al.*, 1979; Turner *et al.*, 1980) assigned a staff member to each patient on a 24-hour basis, using distraction, cajoling, and so forth to prevent the patient from performing his or her compulsions. A somewhat less stringent regimen was employed by Foa and her colleagues (e.g., Foa & Goldstein, 1978; Foa, Steketee, & Milby, 1980). Patients were instructed to refrain from ritualizing, and a relative and/or hospital staff member was asked to be alert to any infractions and to assist the patient in following the instructions. Merely requesting the patient to refrain from ritualizing consituted the response-prevention procedure used in England (e.g., Rachman *et al.*, 1973), in Holland (e.g., Emmelkamp & Kraanen, 1977) and in Greece (Rabavilas *et al.*, 1976).

The effect of supervised response prevention versus mere instructions to refrain from ritualizing was studied systematically with five obsessive-compulsive washers (Mills, Agras, Barlow, & Mills, 1973). Instructions were effective in reducing compulsions, but complete elimination of the rituals was not obtained until strict supervised response prevention was implemented. Indeed, most of the failures reported by Rachman *et al.* (1973) and Marks *et al.* (1975) were attributed to negligence on the part of patients in complying with response-prevention instructions. It seems, then, that although strict supervision may not be necessary for most patients, it may facilitate their adherence to the treatment regimen for some and may result in a more complete elimination of ritualistic behavior.

Differential Effects of Exposure and Response Prevention

As is apparent by now, exposure and response prevention have almost exclusively been employed in tandem. Thus, the separate effect of each procedure could not be ascertained. The question of the differential effect has both clinical and theoretical implications. Because this treatment program is stressful, it is important to ascertain whether exposure and response prevention must both be applied. Theoretically, the differential effect of exposure and response prevention bear on the two-stage theory of fear and avoidance described earlier. This model suggests the need for implementation of anxiety-reduction procedures such as prolonged exposure.* Because ritualistic behavior terminates confrontation with the anxiety-evoking stimuli, its emission should be blocked to permit prolonged exposure to occur.

Does response prevention serve merely to prolong exposure and in this way to eliminate the anxiety and the urge to engage in compulsive behavior, as suggested by Marks (1980)? Negating this proposition are observations that anxiety may be eliminated; yet compulsive behavior persists (Marks et al., 1969; Walton & Mather, 1963). Perhaps, then, exposure and response prevention operate through separate mechanisms, both of which are required to reduce obsessive-compulsive symptoms successfully.

*Prolonged exposure has been found to result in reduction of anxiety responses, both subjective and physiological (Foa & Chambless, 1978; Grayson, Foa, & Steketee, 1982; Nune & Marks, 1975).

From a series of five single-case studies, Mills, *et al.* (1973) found that response prevention alone virtually eliminated ritualistic behavior, whereas exposure alone resulted in either no change or in an increase in compulsions and subjective urges to ritualize. However, contact with the discomfort-evoking stimuli was short, and thus the patients may not have received adequate exposure. Indeed, as reported earlier, brief exposure was demonstrated to be less effective than prolonged exposure. In another series of single-case experiments, Turner *et al.* (1979) found further support for the preceding results. Response prevention ameliorated ritualistic behavior, but the addition of exposure did not further reduce them. Unfortunately, no measure of anxiety was reported for this subject, so the effect of exposure and response prevention on it could not be assessed. In a second case, response prevention again reduced rituals, and flooding did not result in an additional decrease; as to anxiety, some reduction was evident during response prevention with further amelioration resulting from flooding. In a second series of single-case studies, Turner *et al.* (1980) observed that in one patient, flooding alone did not affect compulsive behavior, but neither did response prevention. The authors commented, however, that the patient was considerably depressed and anxious. As we shall see later, depression may be a hindrance to the effectiveness of behavioral treatment and thus may account for the impotence of the two procedures. In yet another case, response prevention affected ritualistic behavior but not anxiety.

In additional attempt to delineate the separate and combined impact of exposure and response prevention, Lipsedge (1974) planned to carry out a crossover design, in which response prevention would be contrasted with continuation of rituals and with a no treatment control condition. The study was not completed. However, the data that were collected seemed to suggest that mere exposure resulted in only slight improvement in ritualistic behavior, substantially less than that obtained by response prevention. In contrast to the results obtained in the single-case experiments noted before, Lipsedge found that response prevention was more effective in reducing anxiety than was exposure.

Further data on the differential effects of exposure and response prevention was obtained by Foa and her colleagues. In the first experiment, Foa, Steketee, and Milby (1980) employed a crossover design. Eight patients were randomly assigned to the following two treatment groups: exposure alone followed by exposure and response prevention (Group A); response prevention alone followed by the combined treatment (Group B). Treatment consisted of two periods of 10 daily 2-hour sessions, separated by 4 days during which patients were requested to record their washing behavior. Exposure-only treatment included deliberate contact with the discomfort-evoking stimuli; 4 additional hours of exposure were assigned as homework. Patients were allowed to ritualize as they wished during the 6 hours of exposure, but after each washing they were immediately recontaminated. Response-prevention treatment consisted of strict blocking of ritualistic cleaning and washing; no contact with water was allowed throughout treatment, with the exception of one supervised 10-minute shower every fifth day. Patients were allowed to avoid contact with contaminants, and no deliberate exposure was implemented. During the second phase of the experiment, both groups received a combination of exposure and response prevention for an additional 10 sessions (2 weeks).

To assess the effectiveness of each treatment modality, time spent ritualizing and subjective anxiety/discomfort to the most feared contaminant were recorded. After the first phase, the group who received response prevention only washed significantly less than did the group receiving exposure only. This difference disappeared by the third assessment after response prevention was implemented for the latter group (see Figure 4). With regard to subjective anxiety, the group who received exposure only reported significantly less discomfort when in contact with the worst contaminant than did the group who received response prevention only. After the ad-

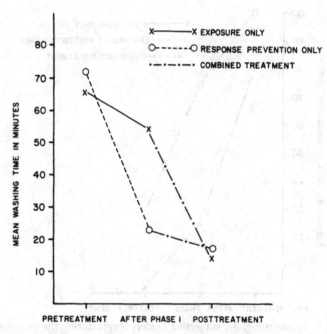

FIGURE 4. Mean washing time for treatment by exposure only, by response prevention only, and by the combination of the two. From "Differential Effects of Exposure and Response Prevention in Obsessive-Compulsive Washers" by E.B. Foa, G. Steketee, and J.B. Milby, 1980, *Journal of Consulting and Clinical Psychology, 48,* p. 73. Copyright 1980. Reprinted by permission.

dition of prolonged exposure, the latter group again did not
differ from the former; both showed significant reduction in
subjective anxiety. These results are depicted in Figure 5.
These findings indicate that exposure affected anxiety to contaminants more than did response prevention. Rituals, on the
other hand, were reduced more by response prevention than
by exposure. When the omitted procedure was added during

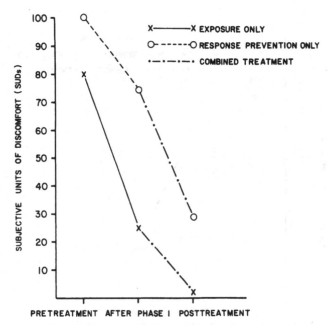

FIGURE 5. Mean highest subjective anxiety levels during the exposure
test for treatments by exposure only, by response prevention only,
and by a combination of the two. From "Differential Effects of Exposure and Response Prevention in Obsessive-Compulsive Washers"
by E.B. Foa, G. Steketee, and J.B. Milby, 1980, *Journal of Consulting
and Clinical Psychology, 48*, p. 74. Copyright 1980. Reprinted by permission.

the second phase, the differences between the groups on both anxiety and compulsive behavior disappeared.

Although these results suggest the superiority of the combined treatment over its single components, it is possible that 4 weeks of exposure alone or of response prevention alone would have yielded an outcome equivalent to that obtained following the combined procedure. Therefore, a second study was conducted in which 18 obsessive-compulsive washers were randomly assigned to three treatment groups: exposure *in vivo* alone, response prevention alone, or the combination (Steketee *et al.* 1982). Therapy procedures were identical to those described previously except that all subjects in this experiment received one procedure only for 15 sessions. The measures were the same as those reported before. The results of the experiment are depicted in Figure 6. As expected, exposure alone affected rituals less than did treatment that included response prevention. With regard to subjective anxiety to contaminants, mean scores at posttreatment were calculated separately for each group. These are presented in Figure 7. As in the previous study, anxiety to contaminants was reduced mainly by exposure, whereas ritualistic behavior was affected more by response prevention. Thus, separate mechanisms appear to operate in the two treatment modalities. What are they?

We propose that rituals are maintained not only because they reduce discomfort to contaminants, but also because they are associated with environmental cues (e.g., sinks, bathrooms, water faucets), as well as with internal mood states. It is commonly observed that depressed mood and anxiety prompted by sources other than contaminants may elicit ritualistic behavior. During response prevention, these extraneous cues continue to exist, but because washing is not permitted, they become dissociated from the compulsive be-

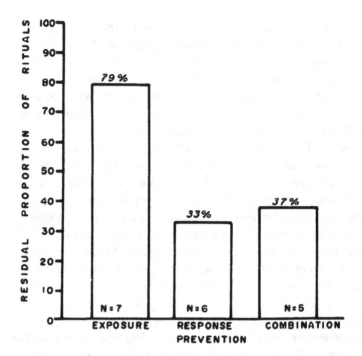

FIGURE 6. Mean residual percentage of rituals for treatment by exposure only, by response prevention only, and by a combination of
the two.

havior and can then be followed by more adaptive responses.

If compulsions are escape behaviors that terminate contact with contaminants, then one would expect that preventing them would prolong accidental exposure to contaminants
and thereby effect reduction of discomfort. Yet, we found that
deliberate exposure was necessary for substantial amelioration
of anxiety to occur. Why? To some extent, obsessive-
compulsives succeed in passively avoiding their feared contaminants. This tendency to avoid is usually augmented during response prevention, thus impeding accidental exposures.

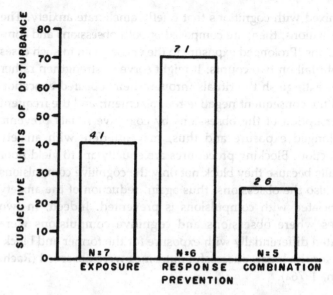

FIGURE 7. Mean subjective anxiety levels after treatment by exposure, by response prevention only, and by a combination of the two.

On the other hand, if, during response prevention alone, patients are motivated to expose themselves deliberately (and face contaminants courageously), anxiety will eventually decrease, and their ability to refrain from ritualizing will persist. Thus, when refraining from rituals is accomplished only through extensive avoidance of feared situations, anxiety will remain high, and a recurrence of compulsive behavior is likely to occur.

If exposure reduces obsessions in ritualizers, why has it yielded inferior results with ruminators? The obsessions of ruminators appear more frequently to be cognitive compulsions than the obsessions of those who have developed motoric rituals. This is to say that anxiety-evoking obsessive material is mixed with cognitions that briefly ameliorate anxiety. The ruminations, then, are composed of both obsessions and compulsions. Prolonged exposure to the entire chain in such cases might fail on two counts: It might serve to strengthen rather than extinguish the rituals through their repeated evocation and the consequent negative reinforcement; and the frequent interruption of the obsessions by cognitive rituals prevents prolonged exposure and thus, may interfere with anxiety reduction. Blocking procedures are equally apt to yield poor results because they block not only the cognitive compulsions but also the obsessions; thus again, reduction of the anxiety associated with compulsions is prevented. Indeed, in two cases where obsessions and cognitive compulsions were treated differentially with exposure for the former and blocking for the latter, successful outcomes were observed (Rachman, 1976a).

Classification and Treatment

The foregoing review of the classification and treatment of obsessionals and ritualizers suggests a unified conceptual framework in which treatment and nosology are related. This relationship between the obsessive-compulsive manifestations and potentially effective treatment interventions for each is given in Table 2.

As is apparent from inspection of the table, we propose that anxiety-evoking cues (obsessions) require exposure techniques, whereas anxiety-reducing responses (rituals) call for blocking procedures. Within these broad categories the exact intervention will vary according to the specific type of symptomatology. The reduction of anxiety generated by external cues is best achieved by exposure *in vivo*; fear of disastrous consequences may call for imaginal exposure. Overt rituals are most adequately controlled by response prevention, and covert rituals may be diminished with the use of blocking techniques intense enough to suppress them, such as electrical shock, thought stopping, or rubber-band snapping. In planning the appropriate treatment program, a careful analysis must be conducted to elucidate external cues and fears of disastrous consequences and to differentiate obsessions from cognitive rituals. Although it is obvious from the preceding discusion that a distinction between obsessions and cognitive rituals is essential for a successful outcome, only Rachman (1976b, 1978) has addressed this issue. This omission hinders a precise evaluation of the various reports on treatment effects in the literature.

Processes during Exposure

The mechanisms that seem to explain the effectiveness of response prevention have been discussed previously. Treatment by exposure has been found to result in reduction of anxiety. What are the processes involved in this change? To study the pattern of anxiety decrement, Lang's (1967) conceptualization of fear as being comprised of three imperfectly correlated components—subjective, physiological, and behavioral—seems fruitful. Using this model, response decrement (habituation), both within and between exposure sessions, was observed. These will be discussed next.

Habituation within Sessions. Observing phobics during *in vivo* exposure, Nune and Marks (1975), Stern and Marks (1973), and Watson, Gaind, and Marks (1972) found that heart rate acceleration habituated within sessions. Similar patterns of heart reduction during *in vivo* exposure were found with obsessive-compulsive washers (Grayson, Foa, & Steketee,

TABLE 2. The Relationship between Obsessive-Compulsive Manifestations and Treatment Interventions

| | Obsessive-compulsive manifestations | | | | |
| | Anxiety-evoking cues (obsessions) | | | Anxiety-reducing responses (compulsions) | |
Treatment interventions	External	Thoughts, images, impulses	Disastrous consequences	Behavioral	Cognitive
Exposure procedures	Prolonged exposure *in vivo*	Imaginal flooding	Imaginal (implosion)		
	Desensitization in vivo	*Systematic desensitization*	*Aversion relief*		
	Exposure with paradoxical relief	Aversion relief	Satiation		

Thought stopping

Aversion by shock

Aversion by rubber band

Alpha wave production

Blank mind

Response prevention

Paradoxical intention

Paradoxical intention

satiation

instruction

Blocking procedures

1982). In this study, 16 patients were exposed to contaminants under distraction and attention-focusing conditions. A balanced design was employed in which subjects were treated with each procedure for one 90-minute session. Habituation of heart rate and of subjective anxiety was observed under both conditions; the rate of response decrement remained constant throughout the exposure period. Within-session habituation was also reported by Shahar and Marks (1980) for heart rate and subjective anxiety and by Foa, Grayson, and Steketee (1982) who measured subjective anxiety only.

There is some evidence that subjective urges to ritualize also habituate following exposure; most of the reduction takes place during the first half-hour (Rachman, de Silva, & Roper, 1976). In a subsequent study, Likierman and Rachman (1980) investigated decrement of both urges to wash and discomfort during six consecutive sessions, each consisting of a single brief exposure followed by a period of 3 hours of response prevention. In all sessions, decrements in subjective discomfort and urges to ritualize were observed, with faster reduction evident in later sessions. Discomfort decreased more rapidly than urges to wash in the first few sessions, thus suggesting a desynchrony between these two subjective phenomena. Likierman and Rachman also noted that initial levels of discomfort and urges to ritualize were higher than those reported in the study by Rachman et al. (1976) and that a longer period of time in the first session was required for these to decline. Moreover, they remained at a higher level following the conclusion of that session. These results suggest a negative relationship between initial level of discomfort and rate of habituation. Further evidence for the impact of the initial intensity of anxiety on habituation within sessions comes from a study by Foa, et al. (1982) in which they found a significant negative correlation (-.33) between these two variables.

When exposure was delivered imaginally, similar patterns of response decrement were observed for heart rate in phobics (Borkovec, 1972; Mathews & Shaw, 1973) and for subjective anxiety in both obsessive-compulsives and agoraphobics (Foa & Chambless, 1978). Response decrements on several subjective indicants of anxiety were also found following short repeated presentation of intrusive thoughts in normal subjects (Parkinson & Rachman, 1980).

Habituation between Sessions. A decrement in anxiety has been observed not only within but also across sessions. Habituation between sessions can be defined in several ways: (a) the difference between the initial level of one session and the initial level of the next; (b) the difference between the final level of the first session and the initial level of the next; or (c) the difference between the final level of one session and that of the next. In studying this phenomenon with two obsessive-compulsives, Shahar and Marks (1980) observed marked reduction of heart rate and subjective anxiety across sessions, when both the beginnings and ends of the two exposure periods were compared. A similar picture was found by Grayson *et al.* (1982) when the difference between initial levels of both heart rate and subjective measures. This measure was preferred because it is not confounded by the degree of within-session habituation. Figures 8 and 9 illustrate these findings. As reflected in these figures, between-session habituation was much greater when a session in which attention was focused on the feared object preceded a session in which the patient was distracted. Thus, either distraction hinders habituation between sessions, or attention focusing facilitates it, or both. Because the crossover design of this study did not permit examination of this issue, a study is currently being conducted in which each patient will receive only one of these two conditions.

E. B. FOA ET AL.

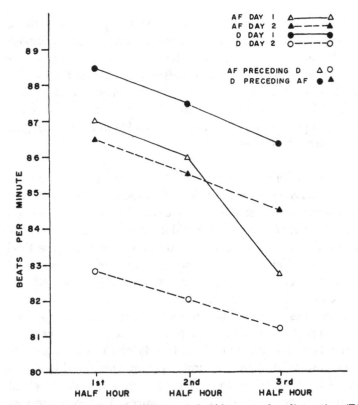

FIGURE 8. Mean heart rate for each half hour under distracting (D) and attention-focusing (AF) conditions.

There was little evidence of any between-session habituation for urges and subjective discomfort in the Likierman and Rachman study when initial levels were compared. However, the degree of anxiety at the end of the first session was much higher than that observed in subsequent sessions. The discrepancy between these findings and those obtained by Shahar and Marks (1980) and Grayson et al. (1982) might be due to the fact that in the former study, subjects received only

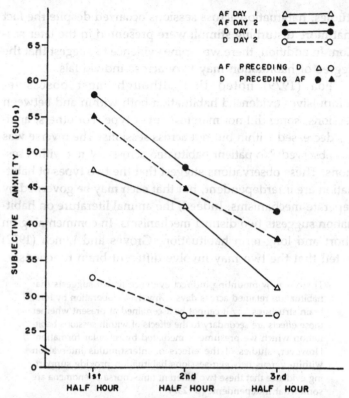

FIGURE 9. Mean subjective anxiety ratings for each half hour under distracting (D) and attention-focusing (AF) conditions.

brief exposure, whereas in the latter one patients were continuously exposed for prolonged periods to the feared stimulus.

In analyzing the subjective reports of anxiety of 22 obsessive-compulsives treated with *in vivo* exposure, Foa *et al.* (1982) found significant response decrements between the beginning of the third and tenth sessions. Similar results were reported by Foa and Chambless (1978) for imaginal exposure. In both

studies, habituation across sessions occurred despite the fact
that more disturbing stimuli were presented in the later session. In addition, there was some evidence to suggest that the
degree of habituation may vary across individuals.

Foa (1979) noted that although most obsessive-
compulsives evidenced habituation both within and between
sessions, some did not manifest either type. For others, anxiety decreased within but not across sessions. The reverse was
not observed: No patient habituated across but not within sessions. These observations suggest that the two types of habituation are interdependent, but that each may be governed by
separate mechanisms. Indeed, the animal literature on habituation suggests two distinct mechanisms. In commentaing on
short and long-term habituation, Groves and Lynch (1972)
noted that the two may involve different brain functions:

> There is now mounting indirect evidence which suggests that
> habituation retained across days...involves elaboration by fore-
> brain structures.... It cannot be ascertained at present whether
> these effects are secondary to the effects of within-sessions habit-
> uation which we presume is mediated by reticular formation.
> However, studies of the effects of interstimulus interval on
> within- versus between-sessions habituation provide support-
> ing evidence that these two different time-course phenomena are
> somewhat independent. (p. 237)

It may be, then, that the reduction of fear within sessions involves the autonomic nervous system, whereas long-term
habituation is influenced more by cognitive processes.

Reactivity, Habituation, and Treatment Outcome. The ability
to habituate has long been implicated as playing a crucial role
in the diminution of fear following exposure treatments. Lader
and Wing (1966) found that complex phobics (agoraphobics,
social phobics, persons with anxiety states, etc.) were more
aroused (as evidenced by more spontaneous fluctuations,

higher skin conductance level, and higher pulse rate) and habituated more slowly than did simple phobics; the latter, in turn, were more aroused and habituated more slowly than did normals. These results have been replicated with other populations differing in anxiety levels (Katkin & McCubbin, 1969; Lykken & Venables, 1971). Lader, Gelder, and Marks (1967) found that patients who did not habituate to tones benefited less from desensitization. Taken together, these findings suggest that both the degree of arousal and capacity to habituate play a role in the outcome of exposure treatments. Further support for this contention is derived from a study by Lang, Melamed, and Hart (1970) who found that a decrement in heart rate and in self-report of fear duing desensitization predicted positive outcome in phobics. In studying the relationship between outcome, depression, and habituation of subjective discomfort within and between sessions, Foa, Grayson, Steketee, and Doppelt (1983a) found that depressed patients habituated less and gained less from treatment. Moreover, when the responses of 50 obsessive-compulsives were analyzed, regardless of their level of depression, habituation within session was related to between-sessions habituation, which in turn was found associated with treatment outcome. If within-session habituation is governed by autonomic processes and habituation between sessions by cognitive ones, then these results suggest that the former precede the latter.

In further exploring process variables during exposure treatment, Foa et al. (1983a) observed that the degree of habituation within and between-sessions was mediated by the intensity of the anxiety response (reactivity) to the most feared item; the greater the initial subjective fear, the less the patients habituated. These results are congruent with those found by Grey, Sartory, and Rachman (1979) in studying phobic subjects. These authors found that subjects who were exposed to situations that aroused moderate anxiety evidenced greater habituation of subjective anxiety than did those exposed to highly disturbing situations. Other investigators have observed that high intensity stimuli appear to hinder habituation in animals (Davis & Wagner, 1969; Groves & Thompson, 1970), as well as in humans (Grayson, 1982; O'Gorman & Jamieson, 1975).

The previously mentioned findings appear to be at odds with the results obtained by Lang et al. (1970). In this study, subjects who evidenced greater reactivity on physiological measures habituated more than did those who were less responsive to feared stimuli. However, in this investigation, subjects who were classified as "highly reactive" were volunteers and may not have been as aroused as the group of patients treated by Foa and her colleagues. In attempting to reconcile these findings, we suggest that perhaps habituation is best facilitated by moderate levels of anxiety because excessive arousal may interfere with the processing of emotional information and low arousal may signal absence of functional exposure (e.g., cognitive avoidance).

The preceding discussion suggests that in planning exposure treatments, attempts should be made to increase the reactivity of avoiders and decrease the arousal level of overreactors. The techniques used to regulate arousal levels will probably vary from one patient to the next. For example, excessive reactors might receive exposure with distraction, whereas low reactors might be treated with an attention-focusing procedure. Other techniques, such as relaxation prior to exposure, might also be employed (Rachman, 1980). Clomipramine has been found helpful in enhancing the effects of behavioral treatment with depressed obsessive-compulsives (Marks et al., 1980). Perhaps this drug promotes habituation by decreasing initial reactivity to discomforting stimuli.

Whether other forms of pharmacologic interventions (e.g., antianxiety agents) will also be of help is as yet undetermined.

In this section we have discussed the relationship between initial reactivity, habituation within sessions, habituation between sessions, and treatment outcome. These three variables appear to be related to mechanisms that operate during exposure. Obviously, a process as complex as fear reduction will be governed by more than these few factors. Other variables that impact on treatment outcome are discussed next.

Success and Failure with Exposure and Response Prevention

Treatment by exposure and response prevention benefits about 75% of the obsessive-compulsives who undergo it, but 25% are unaffected. In discussing their failures, Rachman and Hodgson (1980) note:

> The first and most common [reason], it seems, is inability or unwillingness on the part of the patient to suspend or delay carrying out his or her rituals. The second type of failure arises from inability to tolerate the stress of the exposure treatment sessions. (p. 327)

These observations are congruent with our finding that partial treatment by either exposure or response prevention only is inferior: Patients who do not adhere to the procedural requirements of treatment are, in fact, receiving only partial treatment. But nonadherents are even more likely to fail because their noncommitment may reflect other factors that may impede success (e.g., low expectancy).

It is clear why those who are not committed to treatment do not benefit from it. A more serious conceptual problem arises when we attempt to explain failure among patients who earnestly comply with treatment. What accounts for their failure, and in what way do those who fail differ from those who benefit? Efforts by Hodgson *et al.* (1972) to identify prognostic variables were not very fruitful. By contrast, in a sample of 72 patients, Foa, Grayson, Steketee, and Doppelt (1983a) found several characteristics to be associated with outcome.

Factors Related to Obsessive-Compulsive Symptomatology. One would expect that the longer a patient has engaged in compulsive behavior and the more he or she is limited by these behaviors (i.e., the greater the severity of symptomatology), the stronger should be the habit and, thus, the greater its resistance to extinction. Surprisingly, several authors have failed to find a relationship between severity of symptoms and outcome (Boulougouris, 1977; Foa *et al.*, 1983b; Meyer *et al.*, 1974; Rachman, *et al.*, 1973). In most studies, patients had had their symptoms for more than 3 years, and patients with mild severity of symptoms were not included. In a sample with a wider range of severity and duration of symptoms, these two factors might well be associated with outcome.

In contrast to these findings, a high negative correlation between age at symptom onset and outcome at follow-up was reported by Foa, Grayson, Steketee, & Doppelt, (1983a). The younger the individual was when the symptoms began, the more likely he or she was to maintain treatment gains. Becasue neither *duration* of symptoms nor the patients' *age* at the time of treatment was associated with response to treatment, the previously mentioned relationship cannot be explained by these two variables. Perhaps age of symptom onset is associated with maintenance of treatment gains through its relationship to personality variables not yet investigated. Would patients who manifest pathology at an early age show better ability to cope with their symptoms? At this point, no information about these issues is available.

Depression. Several authors have noted that the presence of severe depression hampers the effectiveness of treatment by exposure and response prevention (e.g., Foa, 1979; Foa, Steketee, & Groves, 1979; Marks, 1973, 1977). In his study of 15 patients, Boulougouris (1977) found a high negative correlation between patients' self-ratings of depression and follow-up scores on the Leyton, although no relationship was found between depression and the rating of their primary obsession.

Studies employing pharmacologic intervention provide further support for the proposition that depression impedes the effectiveness of behavioral treatment. Foa *et al.* (1979) treated a severely depressed obsessive-compulsive with exposure and response prevention without success. However, following the introduction of imipramine, a marked reduction in the level of anxiety associated with contaminants was observed. In a controlled study, Marks *et al.* (1980) employed clomipramine or placebo either alone or in conjunction with behavior therapy to treat 40 obsessive-compulsive patients. An overall drug effect was detected. However, in a *post hoc* analysis of the most and least depressed subjects the following results emerged: Clomipramine facilitated the effects of behavioral treatment only in the depressed group. After completion of behavioral treatment, the five severely depressed patients whose depression was ameliorated showed marked reduction of obsessive-compulsive symptomatology and maintained their gains. On the other hand, the five depressed patients whose depression was not reduced benefited little from exposure and response prevention at posttreatment and evidenced nearly complete relapse at follow-up.

In an attempt to account for the poor outcome observed in depressed obsessive-compulsives, Foa (1979) suggested that depression hampers treatment because it interferes with the process of habituation. To test this proposition, Foa *et al.* (1982) divided 47 obsessive-compulsives into three groups according to severity of depression measured by averaged patient's and assessor's ratings. The results showed that highly depressed patients improved less at posttreatment and at follow-up and evinced a greater relapse rate at follow-up than did patients who were less depressed. The same results were found in a later study employing a larger sample of subjects (Foa *et al.*, 1983a). The relationship between habituation and outcome was discussed in the previous section; habituation both within and between sessions has been found related to success in treatment. To test the hypothesis that depressed patients habituate less than do the nondepressed ones, mean degree of habituation of subjective anxiety during exposure sessions was computed for the severely, moderately, and mildly depressed patients (Foa *et al.*, 1982). A trend in the predicted direction was evident. This relationship was found to be mediated by reactivity (i.e., the level of anxiety reported on first presentation of the most feared stimulus). Perhaps, then, depressed patients are less responsive to treatment because their greater reactivity interferes with the process of habituation.

Anxiety. It is often claimed that in neurotic populations measures of anxiety and depression may reflect the same variable. Is anxiety related to outcome in a manner similar to that found for depression? To answer this question, Foa *et al.* (1983b) divided a sample of 72 obsessive-compulsive patients into three groups according to the severity of anxiety as rated by an assessor. As with depression, anxiety was also found to be related to treatment outcome, but the pattern of this relationship was different. Patients who manifested mild anxiety tended to be improved greatly and to retain their gains at follow-up. However, unlike the highly depressed obsessive-compulsives, those with high anxiety did not necessarily fail. Thus, low anxiety facilitated success but high anxiety did not impede it.

Toward a Predictive Model. On the basis of research findings described previously, Foa *et al.* (1983b) developed a predictive model and tested its utility with a path analysis. As evident from this model (see Figure 10), depression affects reactivity, which in turn impacts on habituation. This latter process influences habituation between sessions, which, in turn impacts directly on posttreatment outcome. Outcome at follow-up was influenced by the patients' response at posttreatment. When the type of treatment (partial vs. combined procedures), anxiety, and age of onset were added to the model, a multiple correlation of .70 between posttreatment outcome and its predictors emerged. With respect to outcome at follow-up, a multiple correlation of all predictors was .78, accounting for 61% of the variance. Obviously, this model does not account for all of the factors that influence success or failure in treatment and maintenance of gains. The need to search for additional predictors is evident.

FURTHER CONSIDERATIONS

It is apparent from the foregoing review that *in vivo* exposure to feared situations coupled with prevention of ritualistic responses has improved the prognosis for obsessive-compulsive ritualizers with 75% showing significant gains. For the present, then, this regimen must be considered the treatment of choice for this disorder. Less encouraging are the findings emerging from studies on obsessionals with cogni-

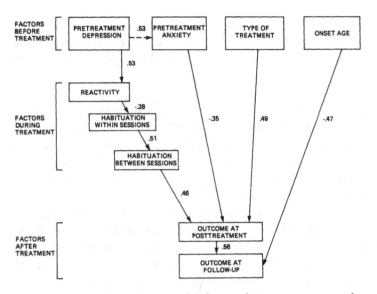

FIGURE 10. A path-analysis model for predicting response to behavioral treatment (exposure and response prevention) of obsessive-
compulsives.

tive compulsions, perhaps because exposure and blocking
procedures have not been appropriately applied in combination. As we have seen with ritualizers, it appears that exposure procedures should be directed at obsessional material,
whereas blocking procedures should be applied to compulsions, whether overt or covert. The omission of either procedure greatly reduces treatment efficacy. In the treatment of obsessionals more often than in that of ritualizers, one procedure
has been omitted, and the one utilized was directed in-
discriminately at both obsessions and cognitive compulsions.
Further research will be needed to determine whether the
combination of exposure and blocking procedures will enhance the outcome with this group of patients.

The past decade has provided us with ample information about the effects of exposure preocedures on a variety of anxiety-based disorders, notably obsessive-compulsive disorder and agoraphobia. Although determination of treatment efficacy has direct implications for the clinical setting, it is crucial to identify the processes that take place during treatment and to study their relationship to specific outcome variables. This line of investigation will enhance our understanding of the mechanisms of fear reduction and fear maintenance, thereby shedding light on why patients succeed or fail in therapy. Such findings will, in turn, lead to changes in treatment procedures and to the development of new, more effective techniques. A most fruitful methodological strategy for such an investigation has been the detailed assessment of the three components of fear: psychophysiological, cognitive, and behavioral. The studies described in this chapter mark a mere beginning in this direction.

One of the processes thought to operate during exposure treatment is habituation of anxiety. There is converging evidence to suggest that a more general capacity to habituate underlies responsiveness to exposure treatment. As noted before, a significant relationship between the rate of habituation to auditory stimuli and response to desensitization has been found. Further, habituation of physiological responses to auditory stimuli and to phobic stimuli during treatment were found related to each other and to fear reduction following exposure (Melamed, 1971). It is of both theoretical and practical interest to investigate further the proposition that a deficit in the ability to habituate to feared stimuli underlies treatment failure and more specifically affects the ability of obsessive-compulsives to benefit from exposure. For example, with regard to habituation and depression, Lader and Wing (1966) found that the rate of habituation of evoked skin conductance responses was greater in normals than in agitated depressed patients. Indirect evidence for a positive relationship between depression and habituation of psychophysiological responses in obsessive-compulsives emerged from a study by Rabavilas, Boulougouris, Perissaki, and Stefanis (1978). They found that ruminators were significantly more depressed than ritualizers, showed greater autonomic reactivity to all stimuli, and habituated more slowly to tones. Is the failure of depressed patients to benefit from treatment due to an impaired capacity to habituate? If so, would reduction of depression enhance habituation? These issues remain to be studied.

Although there is some, albeit scarce, information on the relationship of psychophysiological and subjective anxiety responses to avoidance and escape behaviors (rituals), almost nothing is known about the cognitive changes that take place during or following exposure treatment. When Meyer (1966) first introduced exposure and response-prevention treatment, he entitled his paper, "Modification of Expectations in Cases with Obsessional Rituals," positing the operation of cognitive processes. Specifically, he proposed that when a patient confronts feared stimuli without ritualizing, his or her expectations of consequent disasters are disconfirmed. Additional cognitive changes are suggested by clinical observations of patients who improve. Their self-statements during and between exposure sessions become more positive and their perceived self-efficacy seems to increase during treatment. Such changes do not seem to occur in those who fail.

To date, few efforts to investigate the cognitive changes that take place during and after effective treatment have been attempted. In order to conduct such studies, we must first delineate variables that we hypothesize to be salient. These may include attitudes toward discomfort, judgments of the risks ensuing from contact with the feared stimuli, and perceived helplessness. Although assessment procedures for some of these variables are available, others need to be developed. In the pursuit of investigating the impact of cognitive techniques on obsessive-compulsive symptomatology, Emmelkamp et al. (1980) found cognitive restructuring unhelpful. But perhaps this study was somewhat premature; we must first know what to change before attempting to change it.

The study of habituation patterns and of changes in attitudes and beliefs involved in the treatment of anxiety bear on the wider issue of the relationship between the affective and the cognitive systems. Are the two largely independent of one another, as argued by Zajonc (1980)? Clinical observations suggest not. But what is the nature of the relationship? Do cognitive changes precede, follow, or proceed simultaneously with affective ones? Does the order of change depend on the type of problem (e.g., simple phobias, agoraphobia, obsessive-compulsive neurosis) or on the degree of fear? Is synchrony between psychophysiological and subjective measures of fear related to the degree of cognitive change? These questions only exemplify the breadth of the issues involved in the investigation of anxiety reduction. They also emphasize that the effort to understand the mechanisms involved has barely begun.

REFERENCES

Agras, W. S., Leitenberg, H., Barlow, D. H., Curtis, N., Edwards, J., & Wright, D. Relaxation in systematic desensitization. *Archives of General Psychiatry*, 1971, 25, 511–514.

Akhtar, S., Wig, N. A., Verma, V. K., Pershad, D., & Verma, S. K. A phenomenological analysis of symptoms in obsessive-compulsive neurosis. *British Journal of Psychiatry*, 1975, 127, 342–348.

Barone, D. F., Blum, G. S., & Porter, M. L. Experimental analysis of techniques for eliminating obsessions. *International Journal of Clinical Experimental Hypnosis*, 1975, *23*, 236–248.

Bass, B. A. An unusual behavioral technique for treating obsessive ruminations. *Psychotherapy: Theory, Research and Practice*, 1973, *10*, 191–192.

Baum, M. Extinction of avoidance responding through response prevention (flooding). *Psychological Bulletin*, 1970, *74*, 276–284.

Beech, H. R. Ritualistic activity in obsessional patients. *Journal of Psychosomatic Research*, 1971, *15*, 417–422.

Beech, H. R., & Vaughan, M. *Behavioural treatment of obsessional states.* New York: Wiley, 1978.

Bevan, J. R. Learning theory applied to the treatment of a patient with obsessional ruminations. In H. J. Eysenck (Ed.), *Behaviour therapy and neurosis.* Oxford: Pergamon Press, 1960.

Black, A. The natural history of obsessional neurosis. In H. R. Beech (Ed.), *Obsessional states.* London: Methuen, 1974.

Boersma, K., Den Hengst, S., Dekker, J., & Emmelkamp, P. M. G. Exposure and response prevention: A comparison with obsessive-compulsive patients. *Behaviour Research and Therapy*, 1976, *14*, 19–24.

Borkovec, T. D. Effects of expectancy on the outcome of systematic desensitization and implosive treatments for analogue anxiety. *Behavior Therapy*, 1972, *3*, 29–40.

Boulougouris, J. C. Variables affecting the behaviour modification of obsessive-compulsive patients treated by flooding. In J. C. Boulougouris & A. D. Rabavilas (Eds.), *The treatment of phobic and obsessive-compulsive disorders.* Oxford: Pergamon Press, 1977.

Boulougouris, J. C., & Bassiakos, L. Prolonged flooding in cases with obsessive-compulsive neurosis. *Behaviour Research and Therapy*, 1973, *11*, 227–231.

Boulougouris, J. C., Rabavilas, A. D., & Stefanis, C. Psychophysiological responses in obsessive-compulsive patients. *Behaviour Research and Therapy*, 1977, *15*, 221–230.

Broadhurst, A. It's never too late to learn: An application of conditioned inhibition to obsessional ruminations in an elderly patient. In H. J. Eysenck (Ed.), *Case histories in behavior therapy.* London: Routledge & Kegan Paul, 1976.

Capstick, N., & Seldrup, J. Phenomenological aspects of obsessional patients treated with clomipramine. *British Journal of Psychiatry*, 1973, *122*, 719–720.

Carr, A. T. Compulsive neurosis: Two psychophysiological studies. *Bulletin of the British Psychological Society*, 1971, *24*, 256–257.

Carr, A. T. Compulsive neurosis: A review of the literature. *Psychological Bullentin*, 1974, *81*, 311–318.

Catts, S., & McConaghy, N. Ritual prevention in the treatment of obsessive-compulsive neurosis. *Australian and New Zealand Journal of Psychiatry*, 1975, *9*, 37–41.

Cooper, J. E., Gelder, M. G., & Marks, I. M. Results of behavior therapy in 77 psychiatric patients. *British Medical Journal*, 1965, *1*, 1222-1225.

Davis, M., & Wagner, A. R. Habituation of the startle response under incremental sequence of stimulus intensities. *Journal of Comparative and Physiological Psychology*, 1969, *67*, 486-492.

Dollard, J., & Miller, N. E. *Personality and psychotherapy: An analysis in terms of learning, thinking and culture.* New York: McGraw-Hill, 1950.

Doppelt, H. G. *Personality variables as predictors of treatment outcome of obsessive-compulsives.* Unpublished manuscript, 1981.

Dowson, H. H. The phenomenology of severe obsessive-compulsive neurosis. *British Journal of Psychiatry*, 1977, *131*, 75-78.

Emmelkamp, P. M. G. Self-observation versus flooding in the treatment of agoraphobia. *Behaviour Research and Therapy*, 1974, *12*, 229-237.

Emmelkamp, P. M. G., & Kwee, K. G. Obsessional ruminations: A comparison between thought-stopping and prolonged exposure in imagination. *Behaviour Research and Therapy*, 1977, *15*, 441-444.

Emmelkamp, P. M. G., & van Kraanen, J. Therapist-controlled exposure *in vivo*: A comparison with obsessive-compulsive patients. *Behaviour Research and Therapy*, 1977, *15*, 491-495.

Emmelkamp, P. M. G., & Wessels, H. Flooding in imagination and flooding *in vivo*: A Comparison with agoraphobics. *Behaviour Research and Therapy*, 1975, *13*, 7-15.

Emmelkamp, P. M. G., van der Helm, M., van Zanten, B. L., & Plochy, I. Contributions of self-instructional training to the effectiveness of exposure *in vivo*: A comparison with obsessive-compulsive patients. *Behaviour Research and Therapy*, 1980, *18*, 61-66.

Everaerd, W. F. T., Rijken, H. M., & Emmelkamp, P. M. G. A comparison of "flooding" and successive approximation in the treatment of agoraphobia. *Behaviour Research and Therapy*, 1973, *11*, 105-117.

Farkas, G. M., & Beck, S. Exposure and response prevention of morbid ruminations and compulsive avoidance. *Behaviour Research and Therapy*, 1981, *19*, 257-261.

Foa, E. B. Failure in treating obsessive-compulsives. *Behaviour Research and Therapy*, 1979, *17*, 169-176.

Foa, E. B., & Chambless, D. L. Habituation of subjective anxiety during flooding in imagery. *Behaviour Research and Therapy*, 1978, *16*, 391-399.

Foa, E. B., & Goldstein, A. Continuous exposure and complete response prevention in the treatment of obsessive-compulsive neurosis. *Behavior Therapy*, 1978, *9*, 821-829.

Foa, E. B., & Kozak, M. J. Treatment of anxiety disorders: Implications for psychopathology. In A. H. Tuma & J.D. Maser (Eds.), *Anxiety and the Anxiety Disorders.* Hillsdale, NY: Erlbaum, in press.

Foa, E. B., & Steketee, G. S. Obsessive-compulsives: Conceptual issues and treatment interventions. In M. Hersen, R. M. Eisler, & P. M. Miller (Eds.),

Progress in behavior modification (Vol. 8). New York: Academic Press, 1979.

Foa, E. B., & Tillmanns, A. The treatment of obsessive-compulsive neurosis. In A. Goldstein & E. B. Foa (Eds.), *Handbook of behavioral interventions: A clinical guide.* New York: Wiley, 1980.

Foa, E. B., Steketee, G. S., & Groves, G. A. Use of behavioral therapy and imipramine: A case of obsessive-compulsive neurosis with severe depression. *Behavior Modification*, 1979, *3*, 419–430.

Foa, E. B., Steketee, G., & Milby, J. B. Differential effects of exposure and response prevention in obsessive-compulsive washers. *Journal of Consulting and Clinical Psychology*, 1980, *48*, 71–79.

Foa, E. B., Steketee, G., Turner, R. M., & Fischer, S. C. Effects of imaginal exposure to feared disasters in obsessive-compulsive checkers. *Behaviour Research and Therapy*, 1980, *18*, 449–455.

Foa, E. B., Grayson, J. B., & Steketee, G. Depression, habituation and treatment outcome in obsessive-compulsives. In J. C. Boulougouris (Ed.), *Practical applications of learning theories in psychiatry.* New York: Wiley, 1982.

Foa, E. B., Grayson, J. B., Steketee, G. S., & Doppelt, H. G. Treatment of obsessive-compulsives: When do we fail? In E. B. Foa & P. M. G. Emmelkamp (Eds.), *Failures in behavior therapy.* New York: Wiley, 1983.

Foa, E. B., Grayson, J. B. Steketee, G., Doppelt, H. G., Turner, R. M., & Latimer, P. R. Success and failure in the behavioral treatment of obsessive-compulsives. *Journal of Consulting and Clinical Psychology*, 1983, *51*, 287–297.

Frankl, V. E. Paradoxical intention: A logotherapeutic technique. *American Journal of Psychotherapy*, 1960, *14*, 520–525.

Furst, J. B., & Cooper, A. Failure of systematic desensitization in two cases of obsessive-compulsive neurosis marked by fears of insecticide. *Behaviour Research and Therapy*, 1970, *8*, 203–206.

Gertz, H. O. Experience with the logotherapeutic technique of paradoxical intention in the treatment of phobic and obsessive-compulsive patients. *American Journal of Psychiatry*, 1966, *123*, 548–553.

Grayson, J. B. The elicitation and habituation of orienting and defensive responses to phobic imagery and the incremental stimulus intensity effect. *Psychophysiology*, 1982, *19*, 104–111.

Grayson, J. B., Foa, E. B., & Steketee, G. Habituation during exposure treatment: Distraction versus attention-focusing. *Behavior Therapy and Research*, 1982, *20*, 323–328.

Grey, S. J., Sartory, G., & Rachman, S. Synchronous and desynchronous changes during fear reduction. *Behaviour Research and Therapy*, 1979, *17*, 137–148.

Grimshaw, L. The outcome of obsessional disorder, a follow-up study of 100 cases. *British Journal of Psychiatry*, 1965, *111*, 1051–1056.

Groves, P. M., & Lynch, G. S. Mechanisms of habituation in the brain stem. *Psychological Review*, 1972, *79*, 237–244.

Groves, P. M., & Thompson, R. F. Habituation: A dual-process theory. *Psychological Review*, 1970, 77, 419–450.

Gullick, E. L., & Blanchard, E. B. The use of psychotherapy and behavior therapy in the treatment of an obsessional disorder: An experimental case study. *Journal of Nervous and Mental Disease*, 1973, 156, 427–431.

Haslam, M. T. The treatment of a obsessional patient by reciprocal inhibition. *Behaviour Research and Therapy*, 1965, 2, 213–216.

Haynes, R. Treatment of an obsessive-compulsive checker. *Behaviour Research and Therapy*, 1978, 16, 136–137.

Hodgson, R., & Rachman, S. The effects of contamination and washing in obsessional patients. *Behaviour Research and Therapy*, 1972, 10, 111–117.

Hodgson, R. J., Rachman, S., & Marks, I. M. The treatment of chronic obsessive-compulsive neurosis: Follow-up and further findings. *Behaviour Research and Therapy*, 1972, 10, 181–189.

Hornsveld, R. H. J., Kraaimaat, F. W., & van Dam-Baggen, R. M. J. Anxiety/discomfort and handwashing in obsessive-compulsive and psychiatric control patients. *Behaviour Research and Therapy*, 1979, 17, 223–228.

Janet, P. *Les obsessions et la psychosthenie*. Paris: Bailliere, 1903.

Julien, R. A., Riviere, B., & Note, I. D. Traitement comportemental et cognitif des obsessions et compulsions: résultats et discussion. *Séance du Lundi 27 Octobre*, 1980, 1123–1133.

Katkin, E. S., & McCubbin, R. J. Habituation of the orienting response as a function of individual differences in anxiety and autonomic liability. *Journal of Abnormal Psychology*, 1969, 73, 54–60.

Kazarian, S. S., & Evans, D. R. Modification of obsessional ruminations: A comparative study. *Canadian Journal of Behavioral Science*, 1977, 9, 91–100.

Kenny, F. T., Solyom, L., & Solyom, C. Faradic disruption of obsessive ideation in the treatment of obsessive neurosis. *Behavior Therapy*, 1973, 4, 448–451.

Kenny, F. T., Mowbray, R. M., & Lalani, S. Faradic disruption of obsessive ideation in the treatment of obsessive neurosis: A controlled study. *Behavior Therapy*, 1978, 9, 209–221.

Kringlen, E. Obsessional neurotics, a long term follow-up. *British Journal of Psychiatry*, 1965, 111, 709–722.

Lader, M. H., & Wing, L. Physiological measures, sedative drugs and morbid anxiety. *Maudsley Monograph*. London: Oxford University Press, 1966.

Lader, M. H., Gelder, M. G., & Marks, I. M. Palmar skin conductance measures of predictions of response to desensitization. *Journal of Psychosomatic Research*, 1967, 11, 283–290.

Lang, P. J. Fear reduction and fear behavior: Problems in treating a construct. In J. M. Schlien (Ed.), *Research in psychotherapy* (Vol. 3). Washington: American Psychological Association, 1967.

Lang, P. J. Imagery in therapy: An information processing analysis of fear. *Behavior Therapy*, 1977, 8, 862–886.

Lang, P. J. A bio-informational theory of emotional imagery. *Psychophysiology*, 1979, *16*, 495-512.

Lang, P. J., Melamed, B. G., & Hart, J. A psychophysiological analysis of fear modification using an automated desensitization procedure. *Journal of Abnormal Psychology*, 1970, *76*, 220-234.

Lazarus, A. A. New methods in psychotherapy: A case study. *South African Medical Journal*, 1958, *33*, 660-663.

LeBoeuf, A. An automated aversion device in the treatment of a compulsive handwashing ritual. *Journal of Behavior Therapy and Experimental Psychiatry*, 1974, *5*, 267-270.

Leger, L. A. Spurious and actual improvement in the treatment of preoccupying thoughts by thought-stopping. *British Journal of Social and Clinical Psychology*, 1978, *17*, 373-377.

Lewis, A. Problems of obsessional illness. *Proceedings of the Royal Society of Medicine*, 1935, *29*, 325-336.

Likierman, H., & Rachman, S. J. Spontaneous decay of compulsive urges: Cumulative effects. *Behaviour Research and Therapy*, 1980, *18*, 387-394.

Lipper, S., & Feigenbaum, W. M. Obsessive-compulsive neurosis after viewing the fetus during therapeutic abortion. *American Journal of Psychotherapy*, 1976, *30*, 666-674.

Lipsedge, M. S. *Therapeutic approaches to compulsive rituals: A pilot study.* Unpublished master's thesis, University of London, 1974.

Lykken, D. T., & Venables, P. H. Direct measurement of skin conductance: A proposal for standardization. *Psychophysiology*, 1971, *8*, 656-672.

Mackintosh, N. J. *The psychology of animal learning.* New York: Academic Press, 1974.

Mahoney, M. J. The self-management of covert behavior: A case study. *Behavior Therapy*, 1971, *2*, 575-578.

Marks, I. M. Flooding and allied treatments. In W. S. Agras (Ed.), *Behavior modification: Principles and clinical applications.* Boston: Little, Brown, 1972.

Marks, I. M. New approaches to the treatment of obsessive-compulsive disorders. *Journal of Nervous and Mental Disease*, 1973, *156*, 420-426.

Marks, I. M. Clinical studies in phobic, obsessive-compulsive and allied disorders. In W. S. Agras (Ed.), *Behavior therapy in clinical psychiatry.* Boston: Little, Brown, 1977.

Marks, I. M. Pharmacological and behavioral treatment of obsessive-compulsive disorder. Paper presented at the Annual Meeting of the American Psychopathological Association, Washington, D.C., March, 1980.

Marks, I. M., Crowe, E., Drewe, E., Young, J., & Dewhurst, W. G. Obsessive-compulsive neurosis in identical twins. *British Journal of Psychiatry*, 1969, *15*, 991-998.

Marks, I. M., Hodgson, R., & Rachman, S. Treatment of chronic obsessive-compulsive neurosis *in vivo* exposure, a 2 year follow-up and issues in treatment. *British Journal of Psychiatry,* 1975, *127,* 349–364.

Marks, I. M., Bird, J. & Lindley, P. Behavioural nurse therapists 1978—Developments and implications. *Behavioural Psychotherapy,* 1978, *6,* 25–36.

Marks, I. M., Stern, R. S., Mawson, D., Cobb, J., & McDonald, R. Clomipramine and exposure for obsessive-compulsive rituals. *British Journal of Psychiatry,* 1980, *136,* 1–25.

Mathews, A. M. Psychophysiological approaches to the investigation of desensitization. *Psychological Bulletin,* 1971, *76,* 73–91.

Mathews, A. M., & Shaw, P. Emotional arousal and persuasion effects in flooding. *Behaviour Research and Therapy,* 1973, *11,* 587–598.

Mathews, A. M., Johnston, D. W., Lancashire, M., Munby, M. Shaw, P. M., & Gelder, M. G. Imaginal flooding and exposure to real phobic situations: Treatment outcome with agoraphobic patients. *British Journal of Psychiatry,* 1976, *129,* 362–371.

Mathews, A. M., Gelder, M. G., & Johnston, D. W. *Agoraphobia nature and treatment.* New York: Guilford Press, 1981.

McCarthy, B. W. Short term implosive therapy: Case study. *Psychological Reports,* 1972, *30,* 589–590.

McFall, M. E., & Wollersheim, J. P. Obsessive-compulsive neurosis: A cognitive behavioral formulation and approach to treatment. *Cognitive Therapy and Research,* 1979, *3,* 333–348.

McGuire, R. J., & Vallance, M. Aversion therapy by electric shock: A simple technique. *British Medical Journal,* 1964, *1,* 151–153.

Melamed, B. G. *The role of habituation in systematic desnesitization.* Paper presented at the meeting of the American Psychological Association, Washington, DC, 1971.

Meyer, V. Modification of expectations in cases with obsessional rituals. *Behaviour Research and Therapy,* 1966, *4,* 273–280.

Meyer, V., & Levy R. Modification of behavior in obsessive-compulsive disorders. In H. E. Adams & P. Unikel (Eds.), *Issues and trends in behavior therapy.* Springfield, IL: Charles C Thomas, 1973.

Meyer, V., Levy, R., & Schnurer, A. A behavioral treatment of obsessive-compulsive disorders. In H. R. Beech (Ed.), *Obsessional states.* London: Methuen, 1974.

Meyer, V., Robertson, J., & Tatlow, A. Home treatment of an obsessive-compulsive disorder by response prevention. *Journal of Behavior Therapy and Experimental Psychiatry,* 1975, *6,* 37–38.

Mills, G. K., & Solyom, L. Biofeedback of EEG alpha in the treatment of obsessive ruminations: An exploration. *Journal of Behavior Therapy and Experimental Psychiatry,* 1974, *5,* 37–41.

Mills, H. L., Agras, W. S., Barlow, D. H., & Mills, J. R. Compulsive rituals treated by response prevention. *Archives of General Psychiatry,* 1973, *28,* 524–527.

Mowrer, O. A stimulus-response analysis of anxiety and its role as a reinforcing agent. *Psychological Review,* 1939, *46,* 553–565.

Noonan, J .R. An obsessive-compulsive reaction treated by induced anxiety. *American Journal of Psychotherapy,* 1971, *25,* 293–295.

Nune, J. S., & Marks, I. M. Feedback of true heart rate during exposure *in vivo. Archives of General Psychiatry,* 1975, *32,* 933–936.

O'Gorman, J., & Jamieson, R. The incremental stimulus intensity effect and habituation of autonomic responses in man. *Physiological Psychology,* 1975, *3,* 385–389.

Parkinson, L., & Rachman, S. Are intrusive thoughts subject to habituation? *Behaviour Research and Therapy,* 1980, *18,* 409–418.

Pollitt, J. Discussion: Obsessive-compulsive states (abridged). *Proceedings of the Royal Society of Medicine,* 1956, *49,* 842–845.

Rabavilas, A. D., & Boulougouris, J. C. Physiological accompaniments of ruminations, flooding and thought-stopping in obsessive patients. *Behaviour Research and Therapy,* 1974, *12,* 239–243.

Rabavilas, A. D., Boulougouris, J. C., & Stefanis, C. Duration of flooding sessions in the treatment of obsessive-compulsive patients. *Behaviour Research and Therapy,* 1976, *14,* 349–355.

Rabavilas, A. D., Boulougouris, J. C., & Stefanis, C. Compulsive checking diminished when over-checking instructions were disobeyed. *Journal of Behavior Therapy and Experimental Psychiatry,* 1977, *8,* 111–112.

Rabavilas, A. D., Boulougoris, J. C., Perissaki, D., & Stefanis, C. Psychophysiological differences between ruminations and compulsive acts in obsessive-compulsive neurotics. In J. Obiols, C. Ballus, E. Gonzalez-Monclus, & J. Pujol (Eds.), *Biological Psychiatry Today.* Proceedings of the Second World Congress on Biological Psychiatry. New York: Elsevier North-Holland, 1978.

Rabavilas, A. D., Boulougouris, J. C., & Perissaki, C. Therapist qualities related to outcome with exposure *in vivo* in neurotic patients. *Journal of Behavior Therapy and Experimental Psychiatry,* 1979, *10,* 293–299.

Rachman, S. The modification of obsessions: A new formulation. *Behaviour Research and Therapy,* 1976, *14,* 437–443.

Rachman, S. Obsessional-compulsive checking. *Behaviour Research and Therapy,* 1976, *14,* 269–277.

Rachman, S. The passing of the two stage theory of fear and avoidance: Fresh possibilities. *Behaviour Research and Therapy,* 1976, *14,* 125–131.

Rachman, S. An anatomy of obsessions. *Behavior Analysis Modified,* 1978, *2,* 253–278.

Rachman, S. Emotional processing. *Behaviour Research and Therapy,* 1980, *18,* 51–60.

Rachman, S. & Hodgson, R. *Obsessions and compulsions.* Englewood Cliffs, NJ: Prentice-Hall, 1980.

Rachman, S., Hodgson, R., & Marzillier, J. Treatment of an obsessional-compulsive disorder by modelling. *Behaviour Research and Therapy,* 1970, *8,* 385–392.

Rachman, S., Hodgson, R., & Marks, I. M. The treatment of chronic obsessive-compulsive neurosis. *Behaviour Research and Therapy,* 1971, *9,* 237–247.

Rachman, S., Marks, I. M., & Hodgson, R. The treatment of obsessive-compulsive neurotics by modelling and flooding *in vivo. Behaviour Research and Therapy,* 1973, *11,* 463–471.

Rachman, S., de Silva, P., & Roper, G. The spontaneous decay of compulsive urges. *Behaviour Research and Therapy,* 1976, *14,* 445–453.

Rachman, S. J., Cobb, J., Grey, S., McDonald, B., Mawson, D., Sartory, G. & Stern, R. The behavioural treatment of obsessional-compulsive disorders with and without clomipramine. *Behaviour Research and Therapy,* 1979, *17,* 462–478.

Rackensberger, W., & Feinberg, A. M. Treatment of a severe handwashing compulsion by systematic desensitization: A case report. *Journal of Behavior Therapy and Experimental Psychiatry,* 1972, *3,* 123–127.

Rainey, C. A. An obsessive-compulsive neurosis treated by flooding *in vivo. Journal of Behavior Therapy and Experimental Psychiatry,* 1972, *3,* 117–121.

Roper, G., & Rachman, S. Obsessional-compulsive checking: Experimental replication and development. *Behaviour Research and Therapy,* 1976, *14,* 25–32.

Roper, G., Rachman, S., & Hodgson, R. An experiment on obsessional checking. *Behaviour Research and Therapy,* 1973, *11,* 271–277.

Roper, G., Rachman, S., & Marks, I. M. Passive and participant modelling in exposure treatment of obsessive-compulsive neurotics. *Behaviour Research and Therapy,* 1975, *13,* 271–279.

Rubin, R. D., & Merbaum, M. Self-imposed punishment versus desensitization. In R. D. Rubin, H. Fensterheim, A. A. Lazarus, & C. M. Franks (Eds.), *Advances in behavior therapy, 1969.* New York: Academic Press, 1971.

Schneider, K. Schwangs zustande in schizophrenie. *Archiv für Psychiatrie und Nervenkrankheiten,* 1925, *74,* 93–107.

Scrignar, C. B. Exposure time as the main hierarchy variable. *Journal of Behavior Therapy and Experimental Psychiatry,* 1974, *5,* 153–155.

Shahar, A., & Marks, I. M. Habituation during exposure treatment of compulsive rituals. *Behavior Therapy,* 1980, *11,* 397–401.

Shipley, R. H., Mock, L. A., & Levis, D. J. Effects of several response prevention procedures on activity avoidance responding and conditioned fear in rats. *Journal of Comparative and Physiological Psychology,* 1971, *77,* 256–270.

Solyom, L., & Kingstone, E. An obsessive neurosis following morning glory seed ingestion treated by aversion relief. *Journal of Behavior Therapy and Experimental Psychiatry*, 1973, 4, 293–295.

Solyom, L., Zamanzadeh, D., Ledwidge, B., & Kenny, K. Aversion relief treatment of obsessive neurosis. In R. D. Rubin, J. P. Brady, & J. D. Henderson (Eds.), *Advances in behavior therapy*. New York: Academic Press, 1971.

Solyom, L., Garza-Perez, J., Ledwidge, B. L., & Solyom, C. Paradoxical intention in the treatment of obsessive thoughts: A pilot study. *Comprehensive Psychiatry*, 1972, 13, 291–297.

Stampfl, T. G. Implosive therapy: The theory, the subhuman analogue, the strategy and the technique, Part 1. The theory. In S. G. Armitage (Ed.), *Behavior modification techniques in the treatment of emotional disorders*. Battle Creek: V. A. Publications, 1967.

Stampfl, T. G., & Levis, D. J. Essentials of implosive therapy: A learning-theory-based psychodynamic behavioral therapy. *Journal of Abnormal Psychology*, 1967, 72, 496–503.

Steketee, G., Foa, E. B., & Grayson, J. B. Recent advances in the behavioral treatment of obsessive-compulsives. *Archives of General Psychiatry*, 1982, 39, 1365–1371.

Stern, R. S. Treatment of a case of obsessional neurosis using thought-stopping technique. *British Journal of Psychiatry*, 1970, 117, 441–442.

Stern, R. S. Obsessive thoughts: The problem of therapy. *British Journal of Psychiatry*, 1978, 133, 200–205.

Stern, R. S., & Cobb, J. P. Phenomenology of obsessive-compulsive neurosis. *British Journal of Psychiatry*, 1978, 132, 233–239.

Stern, R. S., & Marks, I. M. Brief and prolonged flooding: A comparison in agoraphobic patients. *Archives of General Psychiatry*, 1973, 28, 270–276.

Stern, R. S., Lipsedge, M. S., & Marks, I. M. Obsessive ruminations: A controlled trial of thought-stopping technique. *Behaviour Research and Therapy*, 1975, 11, 659–662.

Tanner, B. A. A case report on the use of relaxation and systematic desensitization to control multiple compulsive behaviors. *Journal of Behavior Therapy and Experimental Psychiatry*, 1971, 2, 267–272.

Teasdale, Y. D. Learning models of obsessional-compulsive disorder. In H. R. Beech (Ed.), *Obsessional states*. London: Methuen, 1974.

Truax, C. B., & Carkuff, R. R. *Toward effective counseling in psychotherapy: Training and practice*. Chicago: Aldine, 1967.

Turner, S. M., Hersen, M., Bellack, A. S., & Wells, K. C. Behavioral treatment of obsessive-compulsive neurosis. *Behaviour Research and Therapy*, 1979, 17, 95–106.

Turner, S. M., Hersen, M., Bellack, A. S., Andrasik, F., & Capparell, H. V. Behavioral and pharmacological treatment of obsessive-compulsive disorders. *Journal of Nervous and Mental Disease*, 1980, 168, 651–657.

Walton, D. The relevance of learning theory to the treatment of an obsessive-compulsive state. In H. J. Eysenck (Ed.), *Behaviour therapy and the neuroses*. Oxford: Pergamon Press, 1960.

Walton, D., & Mather, M. D. The application of learning principles to the treatment of obsessive-compulsive states in the acute and chronic phases of illness. *Behaviour Research and Therapy*, 1963, *1*, 163–174.

Watson, J. P., Gaind, R., & Marks, I. M. Physiological habituation to continuous phobic stimuli. *Behaviour Research and Therapy*, 1972, *10*, 269–278.

Wickramasekera, I. Desensitization, re-sensitization and desensitization again: A preliminary study. *Journal of Behavior Therapy and Experimental Psychiatry*, 1970, *1*, 257–262.

Wisocki, P. A. Treatment of obsessive-compulsive behavior by covert sensitization and covert reinforcement: A case report. *Journal of Behavior Therapy and Experimental Psychiatry*, 1970, *1*, 233–239.

Wolpe, J. *Psychotherapy by reciprocal inhibition*. Stanford: Stanford University Press, 1958.

Wolpe, J. Behaviour therapy in complex neurotic states. *British Journal of Psychiatry*, 1964, *110*, 28–34.

Worsley, J. L. The causation and treatment of obsessionality. In L. E. Burns & J. L. Worsley (Eds.), *Behaviour therapy in the 1970's*. Bristol: Wright, 1970.

Yamagami, T. Treatment of an obsession by thought-stopping. *Journal of Behavior Therapy and Experimental Psychiatry*, 1971, *2*, 133–135.

Zajonc, R. Feeling and thinking. *American Psychologist*, 1980, *35*, 151–175.

3

Short-Term Dynamic Psychotherapy for Patients Suffering from an Obsessive-Compulsive Disorder

PETER E. SIFNEOS

A CLINICAL CASE

A 24-year-old female college junior came to the psychiatry clinic complaining of an inability to make up her mind whether or not to go to Japan and visit other countries in the Far East with her boyfriend who invited her to accompany him on a business trip. She put it as follows:

> As soon as he mentioned the trip, I became very interested to hear all about his plans, but when I heard that he was inviting me to go along, I felt anxious all of a sudden. Actually, that is

PETER E. SIFNEOS • Professor of Psychiatry, Harvard Medical School, and Associate Director, Department of Psychiatry, Beth Israel Hospital, Boston, Massachusetts 02215.

not absolutely correct because I also felt very thrilled at the thought of accompanying him, but my anxiety increased, I became panicky, and I started to have doubts. Questions came to my mind: "Is he good enough for me?" "Would I be happy with him?" "Will I get bored?" "Would I become attracted to someone else?" "Would I want to have sex with someone else?" "Is he as good a lover as I think?" I went on thinking all these thoughts and my doubts increased. I felt paralyzed. Although I know that all these questions were absurd, because I like Bill and we are thinking of living together, nevertheless I could not get rid of these repetitive thoughts from my mind. In addition, I find myself doing ridiculous acts such as knocking on wood many times. What is so silly about it is the need to knock on wood extra times. I know that I love him; yet I go on performing these foolish acts, and I keep on thinking these idiotic thoughts.

This type of chief complaint is typical of many patients with an acute onset of mild obsessive-compulsive symptomatology who are treated successfully by short-term anxiety-provoking psychotherapy, a kind of psychotherapy rooted primarily on psychoanalytic principles. Its technique will be described in more detail later in this chapter.

Short-term anxiety-provoking psychotherapy (STAPP) is a vigorously active psychodynamic treatment involving the production of insight quickly by exposing the patient's hidden conflicts underlying the symptoms. However, before going on with the description of short-term dynamic psychotherapy for obsessive-compulsive neurotic patients, I am going to say a few words about the very nature of obsessive-compulsive disorder (OCD) from the psychodynamic point of view.

Looking at our female patient's chief complaint, one is struck immediately by the onset of her anxiety, which is associated with her boyfriend's invitation to accompany him on his business trip. This invitation acts as a precipitating factor that suddenly gives rise to an acutely painful state—anxiety.

Questions soon begin to flood her mind, and she obsessively thinks about them without being able to answer them although she recognizes their absurdity. In addition, she is compelled to perform compulsive acts—the knocking on wood—that she considers to be "idiotic" and that, of course, are useless, do not alleviate her anxiety, are totally ineffective, and if anything, seem to paralyze her.

How then can we explain this patient's neurotic behavior pattern psychodynamically? It was Freud (1949), of course, who originated the psychoanalytic theory of the obsessional neuroses by conceiving the presence of an unconscious psychological conflict that he described extensively in his case history of the "rat man." The key to understanding the psychodynamic processes involved was the recognition of the different defense mechanisms that were used in the production of the symptoms.

PSYCHODYNAMIC EXPLANATIONS

The mechanisms that one observes the obsessive-compulsive patient utilizing are the following: regression, isolation, reaction formation, undoing, and displacement (Nemiah 1980).

Regression

Because of predisposing genetic factors existing during childhood, such as, for example, an extreme need for control, perfectionism, cautious thoughtfulness as well as environmental stimuli; regression takes place from the phase where oedipal genital features predominate to an anal sadistic level of personality organization with a resulting preoccupation with anger and dirt. This regression therefore helps the patient avoid genital conflicts and the anxiety that is likely to be experienced as a consequence.

As a result of this regression, magical thinking makes its appearance with marked ambivalence between love and hate and with omnipotent features that complicate the treatment of the obsessive-compulsive neurotic patients. The degree to which these factors exist plays a crucial role as to whether the psychotherapy will succeed or not. If the superstitious narcissistic preoccupation is too extreme, it tends to distort the thinking process to such an extent that a paralyzing incapability to arrive at any kind of decision takes place, and the strong compulsion of doubt makes the therapy almost impossible. If, on the other hand, these features are not rigidly fixed, then an opportunity is given to the therapist to reverse these regressive tendencies, help the patient to face the feelings resulting from the oedipal conflicts, and understand the ineffective ways that he or she has utilized to deal with them.

Reaction Formation

This mechanism of defense tends to emphasize that attitudes that are opposite to the underlying impulses take place and give rise to inappropriate patterns of behavior. If one has a tendency to enjoy hurting people, in order to avoid these wishes, he or she behaves in a passive and masochistic manner, which opposes the desire to enjoy being sadistic.

Isolation

An attempt is made to separate the impulse and the resulting feelings from the thoughts and fantasies that are associated with them by use of isolation. For example, although the patient may talk extensively and have elaborate associations about a very gruesome situation, he or she denies any feelings of anxiety or disgust that would appropriately be associated with it.

Undoing

Undoing is associated primarily with compulsive acts which alter the potential results of the anxiety by producing obsessions. For example, a patient who, as he drove on the highway, observed that a rock was lying on the pavement as he passed it by might have the thought that another driver might hit the rock and have an accident as a result of which he might die. He therefore stops his car, gets out, and walks toward the rock with the intent of throwing it away, but soon he starts thinking that his behavior is silly, and he returns to his car, only to get out again and compulsively repeat this action several times.

Displacement

The tendency to displace feelings on another person or another object that clearly do not belong to them helps the patient to diffuse his or her anxiety and is commonly used by the obsessive-compulsive individual. All these defense mechanisms, in various combinations and degrees of intensity, give rise to the obsessive-compulsive neurosis, the natural history of which, however, is not very well known, and therefore prognostic statements about it cannot be made with any degree of certainty. What is fairly safe to state, however, is that an acute onset has a much better prognosis in contrast to a chronic existence of the symptoms.

PSYCHOTHERAPY

Although there are no adequate outcome research studies on the various therapeutic modalities that have been used to treat obsessive-compulsive neurotics, some general statements can be made. Electric shock, pharmacotherapy, and even leucotomies have been used in some cases with success. However, from my clinical experience, which has been very extensive, it can be stated that psychoanalytic psychotherapies and behavior therapy are the treatments of choice for the obsessive-compulsive disorders. In this chapter, the focus is on psychoanalytic therapies.

Psychoanalytically Oriented Therapies

The psychoanalytic approach involves the encouragement of transference manifestations that enable the therapist to deal with the aggressive and ambivalent impulses, to analyze systematically the defenses, and to achieve, in some cases, impressive symptomatic improvement. Such successes, however, depend entirely on a thorough evaluation of the patients' strengths of character and the selection of appropriate candidates who are likely to respond well to the treatment. This emphasis on choosing appropriate patients has been stressed by the workers in the field of short-term dynamic psychotherapy who have specified criteria for selection very explicitly at the outset and who have continued to work on perfecting them ever since. The techniques of short-term dynamic psychotherapy in reference to obsessive-compulsive disorder will now be discussed in more detail.

The Nature of Short-Term Dynamic or Anxiety-Provoking Psychotherapy

What is obvious from the previous discussion is that one must assess as soon as possible the patient's neurotic difficulties in terms of the following factors: chronicity of the symptoms; rigidity of the defense mechanisms in general and of the prevailing ambivalence in particular; environmental stress; degree of childhood fixation; genetic predisposition; character traits; and, above all, the degree of the regression.

On the basis of these evaluations, one can divide obsessive-compulsive patients into two large groups, which, although they may overlap to some extent, clearly point to completely different directions as far as their basic psychopathology is concerned. These are "chronic obsessive-compulsive neuroses" and "acute obsessive-compulsive neuroses." It is the latter group that seems to respond well to the short-term anxiety-provoking dynamic approach, or STAPP (Sifneos, 1965, 1972, 1979, 1980). STAPP involves a vigorously active technique and emphasizes an interpretative approach by producing insight. This is achieved by systematic exposure of the patient's underlying conflicts, despite the resistances, and even at times by a bypassing of the formidable defense mechanisms, and by interpreting the oedipal wishes. This, of course, produces much anxiety.

There is, in addition to the preceding technical aspects, which will be discussed later in more detail, an educational component to this treatment modality. The therapist becomes an emotionally uninvolved, albeit empathic, teacher. This vital aspect of STAPP appeals greatly to the patient because the joint discoveries that have been made during the sessions encourage him or her to attempt to solve new problems in his or her daily life. These newly acquired problem-solving techniques become an integral part of the patient's character structure and are utilized effectively long after the therapy has come to an end.

The patients who are suffering from acute obsessive-compulsive neuroses are individuals whose interpersonal relations are colored by unresolved oedipal issues and by certain environmental hazards. They usually attempt to avoid their difficulties and resulting anxieties by regressing temporarily to a preoedipal characterological level of personality organization. At such times, they start to utilize inappropriate and ineffective defenses such as reaction formation, undoing, displacement, and isolation that lead to the sudden appearance of symptoms that are unmistakedly obsessive-compulsive in nature. What is striking, however, is a general "fluidity" in both the defenses and the symptoms; in other words, the neurosis does not seem to have solidified into a rigid pattern of behavior. For example, one witnesses the presence of anxiety much more often than one ordinarily encounters in the chronic obsessive patients, indicating that the defense of isolation is not functioning as effectively as it does with the sicker chronic patients. Furthermore, it is this very anxiety that plays a key role in motivating the patient to seek help and offers to him or her the possibility of a successful therapeutic intervention that in some cases can be of relatively short duration. Here is an example.

A 26-year-old female graduate student had developed an acute onset of obsessive thoughts about academic failure after she was given the dates of her oral exams for the defense of her dissertation for a Ph.D. degree in chemistry. She alternated from periods of intense anxiety to periods in which she was calm but totally unable to study effectively. She described that she would constantly think that she would not be able to prepare herself adequately and that she would fail. As she spoke about her potential failure, however, she had a faint smile on her face. When the evaluator pointed to this discrepancy, she said that the thought of a quarrel that she had with her mother came to her mind. She related that she felt irritated with her mother's attempts at reassurance and mentioned that she had told her mother, "Mother, you cannot understand me, and although you are a successful physician, it is clear that you would never have been a successful basic scientist." The patient continued to describe her panic and said that she compulsively took elaborate notes from her books, but when she would realize that they would not serve any useful purpose, she would tear these notes only to find herself feeling more anxious and starting to copy her textbooks all over again. Finally, when her roommate found her awake at 4 A.M. and in tears about her paralyzing symptoms, they talked things over together, and she decided to come to the psychiatric clinic seeking help.

The patient was an only child. She was her father's favorite and said that when she was young, she felt that she would "do anything in the world to please him." Her relationship with her mother was also described as positive, but when she was asked to give an example, she said that she remembered a race with her mother on the beach, and when her mother slipped and fell down, she won. Her father joyfully congratulated her and said that when she grew up she would become a much better athlete than her mother. This pleased her greatly. She did mention also, however, that she admired her mother who was a physician and a teacher at a local medical school and who made a better living than her father who was a commercial artist.

During her puberty, her relationship with her father changed. She felt disgusted by him particularly when he was affectionate with her. She described her father as being seductive with her, which made her feel very uncomfortable, and she related an episode when he confessed to her his dissatisfaction about the sexual relations with his wife. During this time, she felt closer to her mother. At the same time, she felt irritated when her mother gave her a "medical lecture" about the physiology of menstruation and remembered having told her mother that she knew "all about that stuff from her friends" and needed no help from her.

She dated a great deal during high school and college. She had a steady relationship with another student and had satisfactory sexual relations with him, but after 2 years she ended the relationship because she felt that he had become too dependent on her. Another relationship ended also in a similar fashion.

Although she was an excellent student, she was always apprehensive at exam time, tended to procrastinate in preparing her term papers, and felt that her professors had underestimated her knowledge when they invariably gave her high grades. When she entered graduate school, her procrastination increased, the delays in preparing her papers became more numerous, and her anxieties about the preparation of her dissertation became more intense.

The patient was accepted for short-term anxiety-provoking psychotherapy, having been found to meet the selection criteria for this treatment. The focus of her treatment became the theme of competition with her mother. Her "fear of success" was viewed as meaning the defeat of her mother in the academic area. The implications of such a "victory" were considered to have special ramifications in terms of her relationship with her father to whom she felt attracted. She defended herself by denying her wishes for, and by using reaction formation, even felt "disgusted" by him.

During her therapy, it became clear that if she successfully defeated her mother she would eliminate her from the competition and that the road to becoming her "father's mistress," a fantasy that she had ever since early childhood would become a reality. The problem with that solution, however, was that she also loved and admired her mother. The obsessive-compulsive neurosis served her as a compromise.

By failing in her exams, she would not surpass and eliminate her mother, and thus she would not have to express her competitive feelings overtly for her. A *status quo* would be achieved, but its price was too high to pay.

As she gained insight into these conflicts and as she was able to deal adequately with her transference feelings for her male therapist, which were similarly ambivalent as they had been for her father, her symptoms started to decrease. Having obtained an extension for the defense of her thesis, she was able to study, and finally, 3 months later, she passed her exams with flying colors.

Seen 2 years later in a follow-up interview, she was symptom free. She had also moved out from her parents' house, her competition with her mother had disappeared, and she had an excellent job as a chemist with a pharmaceutical company. She was engaged to be married. Thus, it was thought that the basic conflicts underlying her acute obsessive-compulsive disorder had been resolved. The question that should be raised at this point has to do with how to go about discovering this type of individual whose obsessive-compulsive neurotic symptoms will improve with short-term dynamic psychotherapy. The answer to this question is the specification of criteria for selection.

Criteria for Selection

Acute Onset and Crisis Situation. As mentioned already, an acute onset is an easy parameter to use, but there are other dimensions that one should take into consideration. These have to do with the intensity of the painful feelings in general and the anxiety in particular, which has a potential for becoming a crisis. A crisis is a turning point for better or for worse. This impending crisis results from an inability to deal effectively with environmental hazards. The reason for this failure has to do with the utilization of maladaptive defense mechanisms to deal with the anxiety.

Fluidity of Obsessive Defense Mechanisms. Because the anxiety is present, as mentioned already, it is obvious that the obsessive-compulsive defense mechanisms are not functioning very efficiently or rigidly enough, and, this anxiety becomes evident. This gives a golden opportunity for the therapist to take advantage of this inefficient functioning and convince the patient to learn to use more effective ways to deal with the anxiety and its underlying psychological conflicts. This in turn may help the patient overcome the crisis and return to a preexisting state of emotional equilibrium.

Above-Average Psychological Sophistication. Coupled with an above-average intelligence, this capacity connotes an ability to think psychologically and not to expect passively that the therapist will perform some kind of a miracle and magically eliminate the patient's problem.

A "Meaningful" Relationship during Childhood. The documentation of a "good," "altruistic," "give-and-take" kind of interaction, which are all aspects of this "meaningful" relationship with another person, is important because it demonstrates that the patient has had the capability to deal with at least one other human being effectively, and, as a result of this, he or she has learned to deal fairly successfully with the vicissitudes of interpersonal relations.

Motivation for "Change." Motivation not only to receive help and obtain symptom relief but rather, and more importantly, to *change* is an important selection criterion. In addition, it has been demonstrated to have prognostic features for successful outcome, and for this reason we have developed seven additional subcriteria in order to assess it. These are (a) an ability to recognize that the difficulties experienced by the patient are psychological in nature; (b) honesty in reporting about oneself; (c) willingness to participate actively in the psychiatric evaluation; (d) curiosity and introspection about oneself; (e) a basic wish to change; (f) a realistic expectation of the results of the treatment; and (g) a willingness to make a tangible sacrifice.

Interaction with the Evaluator. A flexible ability to interact with the interviewer and express affect during the evaluation session is proof that the patient has indeed learned how to deal with other people, and has mastered the vicissitudes of interpersonal conflicts emanating from complicated human relationships.

Developmental History Taking

In order to ascertain whether indeed the patient does or does not fulfill the preceding criteria for selection, one should take a systematic developmental history that constitutes the second most important part of the evaluation interview.

Dynamic Formulation, Psychotherapeutic Focus, and Agreement

What is left for the therapist to do are two more tasks. First, as a result of the history taking and the fulfillment of the criteria for selection, a dynamic formulation must have been formed in his or her mind that, if focused upon during the subsequent therapy, offers the possibility of a resolution of the patient's difficulties. Once this formulation is arrived at, it must be communicated to the patient, and an agreement must be reached between the two participants that their mutual work will be focused on the resolution of this formulation. At this point the therapeutic work can proceed.

Let us now return to the young female graduate student, who was mentioned previously, to see why she was thought to be a good candidate for short-term dynamic psychotherapy. First, she had a sudden onset of obsessive symptoms and, as a result, she became so anxious that she found herself in a critical situation. As the deadline for her exams was approaching, she became paralyzed, was unable to study, and compulsive acts followed her obsessive thoughts. The psychological defense mechanisms that she utilized were ineffective because they failed to deal adequately with her anxiety. She was highly motivated to change and showed evidence of psychological sophistication, cooperating actively and giving a truthful account of herself. She had realistic expectations of the outcome and was willing to come early in the morning, the only time that was available for her therapy hours. She was aware that her difficulties might be related to her interaction with her parents, but she had been unable to go any further in that direction and thus could not extricate herself from her predicament.

From her history, it was clear that she had several "give-and-take" relations with people, including her father and two girlfriends, one of whom she was still seeing at that time. Despite conflicts with her mother, she nevertheless acknowledged having positive feelings in the form of admiration for her. Actually, the conflicts between the two of them appeared only when there was competition for the affection of father. Her interactions with the evaluator were good. She expressed her feelings openly, honestly, and in a forthright manner.

The therapist, on the basis of the information given to him by the patient, was able to arrive at the following formulation that he communicated to her. He received her agreement to cooperate. The patient was told that, on the basis of what she had narrated, it appeared to the therapist that her attachment to her father gave rise to competitive feelings with her mother over his affection. The fear that if she "succeeded" she might be able to surpass her mother and thus eliminate her from the competition was also verbalized. This victory, however, she was told, would not satisfy her because she loved her mother. She was therefore caught between the horns of a dilemma, which was displaced into the academic arena. Her obsessive-compulsive neurosis pointed clearly to an abortive way to deall with this conflict.

On the basis of all this preliminary work, the therapist was now able to utilize his specialized techniques of short-term dynamic psychotherapy that had been found to be effective in treating these types of patients and that will be described at this point.

THERAPEUTIC TECHNIQUES OF
SHORT-TERM DYNAMIC PSYCHOTHERAPY

Establishment of a Working/Therapeutic Alliance

Although it must be obvious that even during the evaluation interview the evaluator and the patient have worked cooperatively, one of the first technical aspects of this kind of therapy involves the reinforcement of the working alliance to become a therapeutic one as soon as possible, so as to offer the possibility for a "corrective emotional experience" to take place, enabling the patient to solve his or her psychological conflicts (Alexander & French, 1946).

Early Utilization of Positive Transference

Transference manifestations, which for all intents and purposes vary from patient to patient, although ambivalent to
some degree, are predominately in favor of the positive feelings for the therapist, particularly in the early phases of the
treatment. After the therapeutic alliance has been solidified,
the patient feels more secure about his or her interactions with
the therapist and feels free to express more negative and competitive feelings.

A distinction at this point should be made between *transference* and *transference neurosis*. The former, as viewed by
Freud and Glover, is a normal affective phenomenon having
both conscious and unconscious elements that are governed
primarily by the mechanisms of displacement (Freud 1958;
Glover 1955). The transference neurosis that occurs during the
height of the psychoanalysis of the neuroses is a much more
intensive psychological phenomenon, and because of this, its
development must be avoided at all costs. The reason for this
has to do with the inability of the therapist to analyze it in
face-to-face weekly psychotherapy. The dissolution of a transference neurosis can take place only by the psychoanalytic
technique of free association that is unavailable to him or her
in psychotherapy. A way, therefore, to avoid getting entan-
gled with the transference neurosis is to utilize actively the
positive transference that, as mentioned already,
predominates in the early phase of psychotherapy and not to
wait for it to appear as resistance. In this way, the utilization
of the patient's transference becomes the main technical therapeutic tool of short-term dynamic psychotherapy. The reason for this will become obvious during the subsequent discussion about the parent-transference links.

Parent-Transference Links

The ability of the therapist to make connections between experiences and feelings for key people in the patient's past, such as parents, with feelings that are experienced in reference to the therapist enables him or her to create an atmosphere where "a corrective emotional experience" can take place that acts as a powerful motivating force to help the patient abandon his or her neurotic ways of behavior.

Active Concentration on a Central Focus

The psychodynamic hypothesis that was agreed as the point of concentration for both therapist and patient in an effort to resolve the patient's basic problem becomes the main area of work between the two participants and is referred to as the *specified focus*. The work involved in its resolution is referred to as *focalization*. Such foci involve problems of grief reactions, of loss and separation, and in particular, of unresolved oedipal or triangular conflicts. The latter are being investigated extensively by a systematic research study at Harvard at the psychiatry department of the Beth Israel Hospital in Boston.

Staying within the specified focus makes the patient anxious, but the therapist does not have to worry about the development of a serious deterioration. Having evaluated the patient's strengths of character extensively during the evaluation, he or she feels secure about their existence. If anything, he or she utilizes this anxiety to further motivate the patient to look into his or her conflicts and to try to learn to resolve them. He or she actively confronts the patient with paradoxical behavior patterns. He or she clarifies points from the past and connects them with current daily difficulties. By use of clear-cut examples, the therapist can make parent-transference links from information that has been painstakingly collected by him or her from previous interviews. These interpretations enable the patient to reexamine these difficulties in light of the new material that has been amassed.

The oedipal conflict can be easily acknowledged, the wishes and desires can be expressed without a need to hide them, the regressive aspects can be seen as serving the purpose of avoiding the anxiety, the defensive mechanisms that are utilized and that give rise to the obsessive-compulsive symptoms can be understood, and their ineffectiveness can be realized. Finally, the possibility will be offered for the recognition that the problems that the patient encounters in his or her daily life are clearly related to these psychological conflicts around the specified focus which have been brought to the surface with the aid of the therapist.

Avoidance of Pregenital Characterological Issues

Another technical feature of short-term dynamic psychotherapy of obsessive-compulsive neurosis, in addition to the activity involving all the technical aspects that have been described already, lies in avoiding systematically the conflicts relating to pregenital characterological issues that are brought up by the patients as a smoke screen in order not to experience the anxiety that has been aroused as a result of the treatment. This technical maneuver also helps delay the development of the transference neurosis, which, if allowed to become consolidated, will impair the therapy as mentioned already.

Repeated Challenge to the Ambivalence

Because ambivalence is a characteristic feature of the obsessive-compulsive neurotic patient, its repeated demonstration, particularly in the latter part of the therapy where it predominates, serves the purpose of setting the stage for the terminal phase of the treatment, when changes in the patient's attitudes take place and new behavior patterns tend to make their appearance.

Recapitulation and Summary

Periodically, and particularly in the mid- to latter phase of the therapy, the therapist should summarize what has been learned and recapitulate the progress that has been made. The best way to do this is by giving to the patient specific examples rather than making abstract generalizations. These examples have great weight because they do play a role in convincing the patient to give up his or her neurotic ways. At the same time, the therapist should be watching for the appearance of tangible evidence of change taking place. Such changes then can be viewed as earmarks of the development of new attitudes, and therefore the end of the treatment should be considered seriously.

Early Termination of the Treatment

The difficulties about an early termination of psychotherapy are usually rooted in the therapist's educational experiences. Because many trainees have been educated to offer long-term psychotherapy with seriously disturbed patients

and have witnessed the problems that come up at times of termination, which they feel a need to work through, they make
the mistake of expecting that a long terminal phase must also
take place with short-term psychotherapy patients. Furthermore, despite the evidence of change and development of
new attitudes, they tend to doubt their importance and continue to insist that further work with separation issues must
take place. Thus, the inexperienced therapists raise the possibility of examining problems that are not related to the central focus. This attitude not only tends to prolong the treatment unnecessarily, but it also contributes to the probability
that a transference neurosis will develop and an impasse will
be reached. It is therefore imperative that the supervisor be
cognizant of these potential problems and keep pressuring the
student to bring the therapy to an end. Before concluding this
discussion, one should refer to the work of Davanloo (personal communication, 1979) with more chronic obsessive-
compulsive patients, which is referred to as ''broad focused
short-term dynamic psychotherapy.''

The main aspects of his technique involve four specific
phases. At first, the therapist, as has already been mentioned,
must attempt systematically to establish a therapeutic alliance
by use of early clarifications involving transference issues. Following this, a systematic assualt is launched on the patient's
defensive structure until a breaking point is reached. This is
heralded by an appearance of anxiety as well as other feelings
that are encouraged by the therapist to be expressed openly.
Transference interpretations continue to be used actively, and
in the working-through phase the patient is encouraged to understand his or her own psychodynamics. The therapy ends
by a detailed analysis of separation problems. Generally
speaking, Davanloo reports good results with this technique.

Outcome

Although it was originally thought that no basic characterological changes can be expected to take place as a result of short-term dynamic psychotherapy with obsessive-compulsive neurotic patients, more recently, as a result of more systematic long-term follow-up observations, it has become clear that basic changes in the patient's character structure do indeed take place.

What is commonly seen in patients is that:

1. They overcome their psychological crisis.
2. They show new and more adaptive patterns of behavior with considerable evidence of self-understanding.
3. There is evidence of development of new learning and problem solving that is utilized effectively to solve new problems in the patients' everday lives long after the therapy has terminated.
4. They have improved interpersonal relations with key people in their environment.
5. There is considerable decrease in the ambivalence.
6. The obsessive-compulsive symptomatology is greatly diminished.
7. There is evidence of increased self-esteem.
8. They do not feel a need for further therapy and express positive feelings for their therapists whom they view as being instrumental in helping them to overcome their problems.
9. The *specific predisposing factors* underlying their emotional difficulties are resolved or are thought to have improved considerably.

All in all, it can be stated that the short-term dynamic psychotherapeutic techniques can be utilized effectively with well-selected obsessive-compulsive patients. Furthermore, it is also evident that these techniques may be tried with sicker patients.

It must be obvious from this presentation that the emphasis in brief dynamic psychotherapies in general and STAPP in particular has not been on tagging patients with diagnostic labels but rather on dealing with the psychological conflicts underlyiing their emotional difficulties. It is precisely this ability of the therapist to focus actively on these conflicts and on the defense mechanisms that have been utilized during the treatment that produces their resolution and gives rise to a successful outcome. Because of this, it is difficult therefore to give the precise number of obsessive-compulsive patients whom we have treated over the last 25 years. In our first three studies, we treated 627 patients. Approximately 7% to 10% had mild obsessive-compulsive symptomatology.

In our most recent, ongoing research study of STAPP patients with unresolved oedipal conflicts, out of 46 patients, 10 utilized the defense mechanisms that have already been discussed in this chapter and that gave rise, among other problems, to obsessive-compulsive symptoms. These represented 21% of the total. This higher percentage may be due precisely to our concentration on the resolution of only oedipal conflicts rather than other foci such as morbid and grief reactions, separation issues, and the like which we included in our earlier studies.

All 46 patients in our current study are seen in follow-up interviews by one or two independent evaluators to assess the changes that have taken place long after the termination of their treatment.

They are scored on eight points, involving such criteria for outcome as symptoms, interpersonal relations, understanding, problem solving, new learning, work performance, self-esteem, and new attitudes, as well as on the resolution of the specific factors underlying their psychological difficulties.

Scores of 14 to 11 connote a "resolution"; 10 to 7 reveal that the patient is "much improved"; 6 to 3, the patient is viewed as having improved "a little"; and, 2 to -1, the patient is "unchanged" or "worse." The 10 obsessive-compulsive patients scored as follows:

Patient C	score	11.6	
Patient T	score	13	
Patient R	score	13	Resolution
Patient K	score	13.2	
Patient F	score	12.3	
Patient F	score	6.2	
Patient F	score	6	
Patient M	score	8.2	Much improved
Patient H	score	9.1	

One patient withdrew before the end of her therapy and was considered "unchanged." The treatment was viewed as a failure because, despite the efforts of her therapist to motivate her to continue, she claimed that she was feeling better and gave some reasons why she had to leave the area. It was clear, however, that these were excuses, that her motivation had not been assessed correctly, and that the underlying oedipal conflicts had not been resolved.

From all this, it can be concluded that the limit for the use of these short-term dynamic techniques has not been reached as yet, and their future is indeed very promising.

REFERENCES

Alexander, F., & French T. *Psychoanalytic psychotherapy*. New York: Ronald Press, 1946.

Freud, S. A case of obsessional neurosis. *Collected papers* (Vol. III). London: Hogarth Press, 1949.

Freud, S. The dynamics of transference on transference love on beginning treatment. In *The complete psychological works of Sigmund Freud* (Vol. XII). London: Hogarth Press, 1958.

Glover, E. *The technique of psychoanalysis*. New York: International Universities Press, 1955.

Nemiah, J. C. Obsessive compulsive disorder. In *The comprehensive textbook of psychiatry III* (Vol. 2). Baltimore and London: Williams & Wilkins, 1980.

Sifneos, P. E. Seven years experience with short-term psychotherapy, In *Proceedings of the Sixth International Congress of Psychotherapy, Selected lectures*. Basel: S. Karger, 1965.

Sifneos, P. E. *Short-term psychotherapy and emotional crisis*. Cambridge: Harvard University Press, 1972.

Sifneos, P. E. *Short-term dynamic psychotherapy: Evaluation and technique*. New York: Plenum Press, 1979.

Sifneos, P. E. Psychoanalytically oriented short-term dynamic or anxiety provoking psychotherapy for the obsessional neuroses. *The Psychiatric Quarterly*, 1980, 40, 258–271.

4

Comments on the Psychological Treatment of Obsessive-Compulsive Patients

LEON SALZMAN

As a guiding principle, the remediation of emotional disorders requires basic agreements between therapist and patient prior to initiating treatment. Many of these requirements are inimical to the obsessional defensive structure, which tends to make the process of therapy difficult, tedious, and sometimes unrewarding. Although this is notably the case in the psychodynamic approaches, other modalities such as hypnosis, cognitive therapy, and behavioral therapy are also handicapped by the rigidities, avoidance of risk taking, lack of commitment, and related characterological problems of the obsessive-compulsive disorder (OCD) patient. The excessive zeal, which often looks like active cooperation, may, by its

LEON SALZMAN • Georgetown University Medical School, 1800 R Street, NW, Washington, DC 20009.

very intensity, complicate or undermine the therapeutic program. These issues need to be addressed, irrespective of the therapeutic modality. On the other hand, the intricacies and variety of defensive tactics that characterize the human brain are often "played out" in this disorder. Thus, the therapist will have a fascinating and rewarding encounter if he or she can be free, flexible, and open to the complexity of these maneuvers.

The problem facing the therapist, regardless of his or her theoretical orientation, is that of conveying insight and initiating behavioral change without getting caught in the obsessional tug-of-war that is the patient's way of maintaining a rigid style of functioning and avoiding novelty and change. It is paradoxical that in the attempts to clarify an obsessional's life and symptoms, the issues become more complicated and confused. Ordinarily, increasing one's knowledge about a particular problem helps one to focus on the most relevant components. With the OCD patient, however, new issues and qualifications of old ones tend to broaden the inquiry. It often appears as though the patient were deliberately confusing the situation by introducing new issues when there is a real danger of clarifing his or her experiences. By bringing in more details and qualifications, the OCD patient attempts to assure greater accuracy; he or she is trying to be precise and to avoid making errors. The additional factors are generally raised as he or she gets close to seeing his or her responsibility, or even more importantly, his or her failure in some activity. Before the patient is ready to accept an observation about some matter in which he or she played a responsible role, he or she tries to involve every possibility outside himself or herself. Therefore, it looks as if the patient does this purposefully, as these new factors often lead the investigation into a cul-de-sac from which no fruitful return is possible.

The complications, although more apparent in psychodynamic psychotherapy, in the course of which the significance of minor details is traditionally explored, can and do interfere with the process of behavioral analysis and therapy as well. However, it would seem that the more focused approach of behavioral therapists and, indeed, the brand of psychotherapy that was described in detail in the preceding chapter might circumvent some of these complications.

The scholarly overview presented by Rachman clearly illustrates the multifaceted nature of OCD. The etiology, however, is not known, but it would be safe to assume that perhaps genetic and certainly constitutional and environmental factors are at play. Unfortunately, our limited knowledge of the constitutional factors in this disorder does not offer therapeutic guides, and therefore I will limit my comments to the psychological models. These theories can be divided roughly into two categories, namely learning theory and psychodynamic theory. These have been discussed elsewhere in this volume. Hence, instead of attempting a comprehensive review, I would like to briefly present my own conceptualization of the important psychological issues involved and develop a rationale for a therapeutic approach to this complex disorder.

Perhaps the major difference between the two aforementioned modalities lies in the way they view underlying character structure. Whereas behavioral approaches tend to view obsessive-compulsive symptoms as separate from obsessive-compulsive personality, the psychodynamic theories view obsessions and rituals as directly relating to underlying character structure. It is not surprising, therefore, that, as with all neurotic difficulties, the work of psychodynamic psychotherapies has focused on the identification, clarification, and alteration of the characteristic defensive patterns that are thought to maintain the neurosis. Behavior therapy, on the other hand, attempts to alter the clinically significant symptoms directly, believing that a modification of one affects both.

The validity of a therapeutic approach must take into account the goals of therapy. Is the most favorable outcome simply the relief of anxiety, symptom amelioration, increase of productivity, or behavioral or attitudinal change? These goals do not necessarily imply a more superficial expectation in contrast to a deeper, more basic alteration as claimed by some psychoanalytic theorists. The goals may be limited by our present knowledge of the etiology or theoretical differences. It is unfortunate that, in most studies utilizing one modality in contrast to another, these considerations are not stated so that the results can be judged by the expectations instead of by some idealistic, total-cure expectations. If goals are considered, then we might find that the therapy may be extremely effective if limited expectations are the goal, whereas other approaches claiming massive changes may produce only minimal results.

Simply shortening the treatment by insisting on the patient's activity and the active focusing on the problem by the therapist can increase the therapeutic success. In this regard, behavior therapy meets the challenge of the obsessive-compulsive disorders most effectively. It is focused, time limited, and demands that the patients participate and actively work toward change. However, by limiting the cognitive understanding of how the symptom deals with anxiety, it reduces the symptom without necessarily altering the tendency for obsessiveness to be manifested in other areas of living. It is not a matter of symptom substitution that may not occur but the persistence of obsessional traits that can hamper the patient's living. In recent years, behavior therapy has placed increased emphasis on cognitive factors, whereas psychodynamic theory has become less restrained in adopting behavioral tactics in attempting to alter distorted behavior. However, the goals may still differ in spite of the tendency in each modality to compromise long-term goals for short-term gains and vice versa.

Therapy can be defined as the remedial treatment of bodily disorders. It can be specifically classified in many ways, depending upon one's prejudices and preconceptions. There is etiological therapy when the cause of the disorder has been definitely established, in contrast to symptomatic therapy, which is designed to alleviate specific discomforts associated with a disorder. This is the case when isoniazid is used to kill the tubercule bacillus, whereas codeine may be administered to relieve the distressing and disabling cough that accompanies tuberculosis. Thus, some therapies are palliative, but they do not destroy the underlying disorder, whereas others are ameliorative because they undermine and eliminate the causal factor.

Such a significant distinction may be distorted by false claims when etiology is unknown, disputed, or still in the process of being established. This is the case with neuroses, because our definitions and classification are based either on ill-defined etiological factors or behavioral manifestations that may be interpreted in many ways. Therapuetic approaches, therefore, tend to be both palliative and ameliorative. We cannot presently separate those factors because current knowledge of causation is sparse. Behavior therapy, like pharmacotherapy, has the distinct advantage of having known targets and relatively clear effects. Whether it is only palliative and not etiological is still an open question. Psychoanalysis is still based on so many unproven and poorly demonstrated hypotheses that is is more difficult to demonstrate a clear relationship between the process and the alleviation of the disorder or to isolate what elements in the process are ameliorative in contrast to being purely palliative.

The prevailing classification of therapy, beyond the descriptive level of etiologic/symptomatic, conveys value judgments. It expresses the prejudices or preconceptions of the classifier, implying what to him or her is correct or incorrect, true or false, deep or basic, superficial or secondary therapy. How else are we to interpret the labels of deep versus superficial therapy, adjuvant (or subsidiary) versus psychotherapy, or a situation in which all approaches other than the classically defined psychoanalytic techniques are classified as psychotherapy? Often the term *psychotherapy* is used to describe what is thought of as a second-class approach that is nonetiological and therefore, not truly ameliorative. This relects a view of therapy in hierarchical terms. Psychoanalysis or "etiological" therapy is at the top, and all the lesser, nonetiological and therefore symptomatic approaches are on the bottom. Although seemingly attractive and certainly seductive, this viewpoint is destructive and irrational because all valid therapeutic programs reflect varying goals and experiences. There are not simply *pure* versus alloyed methods of treatment. There is a group of descriptive labels that identify the technical processes, such as active versus passive, expressive versus suppressive, and directive versus nondirective approaches.

In my own practice, I utilize a psychotherapeutic approach based on modified psychoanalytic concepts to treat obsessive-compulsive patients. It has been my contention that psychotherapy can be effective, though it is an extremely difficult task because it involves illuminating and exposing the patient's extreme feelings of insecurity and uncertainty that he or she tries to handle through the complicated patterns of defenses. As the patient comes to understand that his or her neurotic structure is a defense against recognizing these weaknesses, he or she can then begin to build a new security system.

At therapy's inception, the obsessional defense cannot be abandoned because the individual is afraid of the consequences. Progress becomes possible when the patient's self-esteem or ego strength becomes sufficiently strengthened to withstand a major assault against these defenses. Although the problems that brought about these defenses are comparatively easy to uncover, the defensive structure that develops around these issues is more difficult to unravel. At times, the particular issues of the patient are obvious and are plainly stated in his or her obsessional ruminations or compulsive rituals. For example, a ritualistic avoidance of knives may be a clear statement within the awareness of the patient that he or she has some uneasiness about losing control of hostile impulses. The identification of the problem, which is the fear of loss of control of hostile impulses, is simple enough. However, it is soon evident that it is not only a fear of injuring someone else that is involved but rather a generalized uneasiness and uncertainty about the possibility of losing control in general or of being, in my opinion, unable to control oneself at all times. The fear of loss of control is the central conflict that gets displaced onto a variety of issues; hostility is an obvious one. Tenderness, however, is often a more significant feeling that needs to be controlled because its presence may leave the person more exposed and threatened by a presumed display of weakness and vulnerability.

As the patient's esteem grows and the awareness of his or her strength increases, he or she can slowly risk abandoning these patterns, thereby freeing him or her to function on a more productive level. The goal is to move from superhuman expectations to human productiveness at whatever level the person is capable of achieving. When the patient recovers, his or her ambitions will no longer be sparked by the neurosis; rather, his or her achievements will be limited only by his or her capacities. The impossible goals that left the patient disappointed will be abandoned. An awareness of a patient's valid capacities to produce may actually stimulate greater activity. In essence, the individual must learn that in abandoning rigid, inflexible patterns of behavior designed to control and protect oneself, the patient can actually feel more secure and capable and can be more productive as well.

The goals and treatment plan for the obessional states can therefore be summarized as follows:

1. To discover and elucidate the basis for the excessive feelings of insecurity that require absolute guarantees before action is pursued.
2. Reduction of symptoms to facilitate relaxation of defenses in an attempt to encourage more adaptive behavior. This can often be done more rapidly with behavioral treatments.
3. To demonstrate by repeated interpretation and encouragement that "guarantees" are not necessary and only interfere with living. This requires active assistance in stimulating new adventures for the patient.
4. To realize that the foregoing is possible only when the patient can acknowledge that anxiety is universal and omnipresent and cannot be permanently eliminated from life.
5. Achievement of a secure and enhanced self-esteem to permit risk taking and abandonment of phobic/compulsive and other distracting activities that would permit direct and responsive behavior. This can be completed through both psychodynamic and behavior modification approaches.

6. Elaboration of the dynamic function of the symptoms and their origins that will enable the patient to attempt some reorganization of his or her behavioral patterns in abandoning the compulsive symptoms.

Goals such as these are achieved through the trust and intimacy that grow out of the therapeutic relationship. However, it also requires skill and intelligence, and the treatment must follow techniques that may differ radically from the classical theoretical models. It is important to (a) avoid strengthening the patient's obsessional tendencies; (b) tailor one's techniques to counter such devices; and (c) to provide a learning experience that may enable the patient to alter his or her defensive patterns. An open, flexible technique with no rigid rules of procedure is demanded, as well as a therapist who is free to experiment and try out modifications in the therapeutic process.

In summary, I believe that our understanding of the obsessive-compulsive disorder requires an integration of psychodynamic and behavior therapies because the resolution of the disabling disorder demands cognitive clarity with behavioral alterations. A rational approach should utilize these modalities because they reinforce rather than weaken the potential for change. The reduction of focus on the rituals through behavior modification may allow clarification of the underlying psychodynamics. The amelioration of a phobia or ritual may so increase the optimistic expectations of further reduction of the obsessional difficulties as to measureably improve the total living.

Can we recommend specific approaches or guidelines for the use of particular modalities? The evidence would indicate that in patients with severe compulsive symptoms, behavioral treatments can be very helpful, whereas psychotherapy might be considered in the milder and less acute cases. On the other hand, the more general obsessive-compulsive characterological differences such as perfectionism, doubting, procrastination, and indecisiveness are best treated, in my opinion, by a psychotherapeutic approach. Presently, there seems to be little evidence of the value of physiological or pharmacological treatments in altering obsessional ruminations. The value of drugs, on the other hand, seems to be related to the anxiety and associated depression present in these disorders.

For the young therapist or novice clinician, we must emphasize the complicated and multifaceted nature of this disorder, even while we focus on particular modalities of therapy. There is no single known cause, and at present no single approach can be accepted without considerable disagreement among well-informed and respected researchers. The most effective tool is an open mind and willingness to utilize the various therapeutic modalities with the aim of enhancing the potential for change. A therapist who can combine both of these psychological approaches in an integrated fashion will be more effective. However, it will not be enough for the behavior therapist to assert that cognitive factors are involved. He or she will need to understand the dynamics of character structure and its role in symptom formation. Conversely, the psychodynamic therapist will need to do more than acknowledge the role of learning and conditioning in human behavior and its dysfunction. He or she will also need to be able to apply these conditioning approaches in his or her therapeutic sessions.

Finally, we must inform patients of the limits of our present therapeutic capacities and understanding of OCD. False promises leading to false hopes, however sincere, can only result in dramatic failure leading to the pursuit of metaphysical and magical therapies that are themselves part of the disease process. The comfort of the patient must be respected, and the search for ultimate causes must be pursued, but we must not demand unreasonable sacrifices to pursue theories that do not have a broad consensus. Rigidity in pursuit of understanding is as obsessional a problem as the disease we are endeavoring to understand and treat.

5

Pharmacotherapy of
Obsessive-Compulsive Disorder

JAMBUR ANANTH

Obsessive-compulsive disorder (OCD) has attracted the attention of many investigators from time immemorial because of the rarity of the disease, the distinctive clinical picture, and the ego-alien nature of the symptoms. Over time, many methods of treatment have been tried, unfortunately, with little success. Thus, pessimism has been generally expressed by many workers regarding the outcome of therapeutic intervention (Kolb, 1968; Lewis, A., 1935; Pollitt, 1957). However, with the progress achieved over the past 20 years in the psychological and somatic treatments of this disorder, there is reason for optimism. Hopefully, the new directions will also provide new insights in the understanding of this crippling disorder. Basic to treatment and evaluation of efficacy are the problems of diagnosis, assessment, and the rationale for treatment.

JAMBUR ANANTH • Director, Psychopharmacology Harbor, UCLA Medical Center, University of California at Los Angeles, Torrance, California 90509.

DIAGNOSIS

At the onset, it appears that the diagnosis of OCD is easy because of the distinctive nature of the illness and its clear-cut history. However, the illness is rare (Goodwin, Guze, & Robins, 1969; Woodruff & Pitts, 1964), and many physicians are not exposed to the illness, which itself poses a diagnostic difficulty. The symptoms occur concomitantly with depression, schizophrenia, borderline syndromes, and organic disorders, including head injury, epilepsy, and Parkinsonism (Brickner, Rosen, & Munro, 1940; Grimshaw, 1965; Schilder, 1938). In addition, infantile autism (Kanner, 1957) has obsessive symptoms as one of the characteristic features. All these resemble OCD, and in some, obsessive symptoms continue to be the dominant psychopathology. Thus, the diagnosis of OCD sometimes is difficult. The results of past studies often are difficult to interpret due to lack of clarity in diagnostic procedures. With the advent of the third edition of the *Diagnostic and Statistical Manual of Mental Disorders* (DSM-III), the criteria for the diagnosis of OCD may have improved. These include the exclusion of Tourette's syndrome, schizophrenia, depression, and organic brain disorder.

Characteristics of obsessive-compulsive symptoms are the following:

1. The obsessional ideas or the compulsion to perform rituals intrudes into consciousness despite the voluntary desire of the person to keep away from them. Thus, they are considered ego alien.
2. The resistance by the person to entertain the idea or perform the ritual produces mounting anxiety. This increasing anxiety itself makes the person yield to the idea or ritual.
3. Performing the ritual's act results in anxiety relief.

Associated with the obsessive syndrome is anxiety and depression. That anxiety plays a predominant role in obsessive disorder has been generally recognized (Rosenberg, 1968). On the other hand, the emotional tone that accompanies obsessions need not be anxiety but can be other unpleasant feelings including anger, discomfort, and specific fear of contamination. Contrary to anxious patients who manifest increased arousal associated with excessive psychomotor activity, obsessive patients may manifest selected slowness in certain activities.

Depression is almost always associated with obsessive disorder. This finding is not surprising as obsessive symptoms are ego alien and disrupt the patient's adjustment. The relationship between depression and obsession is complicated and intriguing. Three possible hypotheses have been put forward: (a) Depression occurs concomitantly with obsessions; (b) depression is secondary to OCD; and (c) OCD is simply an atypical manifestation of depression. Each one of these, though not well substantiated, merits further discussion in view of the series of studies reported by Gittelson (1966a, 1966b, 1966c, 1966d). In this series of publications, she reported that in 52 of the 393 depressed patients included in the sample, frank obsessional symptoms preceded the onset of depressive symptoms. Similarly, Kendell and Discipio (1970) administered the Leyton Obsessive Inventory to a group of 78 depressed patients while depressed and to 72 patients after recovery to assess the relationship between depressive and obsessive symptoms. They noted that there was a significant difference in the symptoms, as well as the resistance scores before and after treatment, indicating the concomitant occurrence of both symptoms. Lewis, as early as 1935, found the presence of obsessional symptoms in 14 of his 61 depressed patients. Thus, it seems that obsessional symptoms do occur during depression.

As an alternative hypothesis, Meyer-Gross, Slater, & Roth (1969) mentioned a rare group of obsessional patients who remit and relapse much the same way as a cyclothymic illness. Other authors (Brown, 1942; Sakai, 1968) reported a genetic relationship between bipolar affective disorders and obsessive-compulsive neurosis, suggesting a link between the two entities. Vanggard (1959) reported OCD manifesting as an episode of endogenous depression. Black (1974) reviewed three studies of the family histories of depression in patients with OCD and noted a positive relationship. All three findings suggest that OCD itself may be a form of depression. On the other hand, occurrence of depression of varying degrees of severity during acute exacerbation of OCD is well known, and the possibility that depression may be the inevitable consequence of the never-ending torture caused by obsessions cannot be ruled out.

ASSESSMENT

There are two aspects of assessment that are of concern to treatment and outcome. They are the natural course of the disorder and the assessment instruments. Without proper assessment instruments, the measurement of the treatment outcome becomes subjective, and without regard to the course of the illness, natural remission may be mistaken for improvement induced by treatment. The natural history of OCD has been reviewed exhaustively by a number of investigators (Black, 1974; Goodwin et al., 1969; Kringlen, 1970). Goodwin et al. (1969) reviewed 13 follow-up studies in seven different countries involving a total of 816 patients. They noted that spontaneous remission of varying duration can occur and that the neurosis is basically a chronic illness. Similar views have been expressed by others (Kalinowsky & Hoch, 1961; Kolb, 1968; Meyer-Gross *et al.*, 1969). In fact, Pollitt (1957) found that 50% of his 81 patients had an episodic course. Some others (Lewis, 1935; Lo, 1967) found episodic courses in 10% to 13% of their patients.

As these reports indicate, the course is not generally episodic, but those with episodic course do affect the assessment of treatment outcome. Basically, a long-term follow-up for at least a year or two is necessary to evaluate treatment efficacy. Second, a randomized placebo group is necessary to minimize the effects of natural remission. Third, a crossover study may assist in substantiating treatment effects in an intrapatient design. Last, it is important to establish whether the treatment is curative, palliative, or even preventive, thereby altering the course of illness.

The measurement of psychopathology is basic to any clinical drug research. Good assessment instruments for OCD have not been available, and therefore many past studies suffered from lack of valid measurement. What do we measure? It is definitely important to measure the anxiety, depression, and obsessive symptoms. Obsessive symptom measurement should include the obsessive ruminations, rituals, phobias (obsessive), and horrific temptations..

Obsessive ruminations are thoughts that intrude into consciousness in spite of resistance by the patient. The patient continues to be absorbed by these thoughts repetitively. A patient of mine would think of why God created the world. At present, I have a patient who ruminates that delirium and craziness are not insanity. This symptom can be distinguished from the forced thought of epilepsy by the fact that the patient resists the obsessive ruminations and not the forced thinking. Also, obsessive ruminations last for hours whereas forced thinking continues for a few minutes. It differs from daydreaming or fantasy, which can be turned off without any anxiety, and it is not repetitive in its content. Obsessive rituals, unlike ruminations, are not mere conceptual entities but motor acts. Typically, the patients perform certain rituals a definite number of times in a particular fashion and sequence. The patients are aware of the irrelevance of their acts, but they carry these acts anyway to obtain relief from anxiety. Quite often, they are embarrassed by their behavior and are tortured by mounting anxiety if they do not perform the rituals. On the other hand, knowing the absurdity of their behavior, they try hard to prevent it. A patient of mine washed her hands compulsively over 100 times and finished a cake of soap daily. When I saw her, the skin of her hands was denuded. Another patient, while walking, had to turn around 180 degrees whenever he came across a manhole on the street. One of my 12-year-old male patients had to turn east and open the blind. When the sun rays came into the room, he would turn north, tap his feet alternately 20 times, bow down to the god 10 times, and eat his breakfast. Another patient, a 30-year-old unmarried male, had to wash his hands five times whenever he touched any food or children.

Obsessive phobias are primarily internal phobias of germs and diseases. Basically, the patients worry about getting contaminated with germs. A 40-year-old wealthy lady had fear of tuberculosis. She was afraid of people coming from the eastern direction as the sanitarium was to the east of her home. She could not live in her home as the door was facing east. Finally, she could not meet or talk with anyone who knew of someone who had had tuberculosis. Obsessive horrific temptations are somewhat infrequent. These are ego-alien urges or impulses to do something bad. A 35-year-old Ceylonese man who came to see me reported an urge to touch electric wries. Another 28-year-old unmarried man was afraid of hurting his girlfriend whenever the dinner table was set and there were knives on the table.

In addition to the measurement of severity of each of these symptoms, it is very useful to list the number of obsessive symptoms and their content. This exercise is not futile. I had a patient with 10 different rituals. After treatment, only 2 rituals continued unabated with the same severity. Unless a symptom count is taken, this patient may be rated as not improved. There are three very useful scales for the measurement of obsessive symptoms. These include the Leyton Obsessive Inventory, the Maudsley Obsessive Compulsive Inventory, and the Philpott Scale.

The Leyton Obsessive Inventory (Cooper, 1970) contains 69 questions dealing with obsessional traits and symptoms. The test is administered by a card-sorting procedure under supervision. The questions included in this questionnaire yield the obsessive trait, the obsessive symptoms, the resistance, and the interference scores. The obsessive trait score measures the premorbid obsessive personality traits, and the obsessive symptom scores measure the obsessive symptoms. Resistance refers to the patient's ability to resist entertaining an idea or performing a ritual. An increase in this score is considered as an indicator of improvement. The interference score provides the degree to which the symptoms interfere with the patient's life. The higher the interference score, the more severe is the sickness. It is so far the most extensively used scale. This scale has been used for the diagnosis of the OCD as well as for measuring changes during treatment (Ananth, Solyom, Bryntwick, & Krishnappa, 1979; Rapoport, Elkins, & Miielsen, 1980; Thoren, Asberg, Cronholm, Jorenstedt, & Traskman, 1980). The difficulties with this scale are that the results are dichotomous (yes or no) and not serial, and hence severity or change (if minimal) cannot be easily measured. The second problem is with the resistance score. Does it decrease or increase with improvement? In our own study (Ananth et al., 1979), the resistance score decreased with improvement. However, Symptom score also had decreased concomitantly. Thus, both a decrease in Resistance score (associated with a moderate to maximum decrease in symptom score) and an increase in resistance score (with minimal change in symptom score) can be indicative of improvement.

The Maudsley Obsessive Compulsive Inventory (Rachman & Hodgson, 1980) is useful in separating subtypes of the obsessive symptoms. Another strategy is to employ graded ratings of an individualized target symptom (Philpott, 1975). In this rating, the number of times a ritual is performed and duration of each ritual are rated. Even obsessive indecision and slowness are quantified by measuring the latency of response. This is a very sensitive index of change, provided the external variable remains unrestricted. Otherwise, changes like locking the washrooms may change shower time to zero and provide false-positive results of improvement.

An assessment of the obsessive-compulsive symptom alone is not sufficient. A severe depression with psychomotor retardation may decrease rituals, which is not indicative of an improvement in OCD. An assessment of value is the employment of standard anxiety and depression scales to indicate the degree of anxiety and depression that are intertwined in the psychopathology of OCD. This is particularly relevant as one can understand the reciprocal relationship between the three groups of symptoms. The assessment of OCD, therefore, requires utilization of a number of rating scales. Simultaneous evaluation of anxiety, depression, and obsessions, along with objective rating of the individual obsessive symptoms, is necessary to assess the efficacy of treatment. Such assessments should be continued for a year to note the dissipation of effect, drug tolerance, side effects, and recurrence of symptoms.

BIOCHEMISTRY

The treatment of any disease can be etiologically or symptomatically oriented. Unfortunately, the etiology of OCD has thus far been elusive. However, certain biochemical abnormalities have been postulated to be associated with this syndrome.

Obsessive compulsions or rituals come under the umbrella of involuntary repetitive movements that include chorea, athetosis, Huntington's chorea, senile dyskinesia, the stereotypies of schizophrenia, and Gilles de la Tourette syndrome. In tardive dyskinesia, Huntington's chorea, and Gilles de la Tourette syndrome, dopaminergic supersensitivity has been hypothesized (Ananth, 1982; Creese, Bivet & Snyder, 1977; Klawan, 1973; Owen, Crow, Foulter, Cross, Longden, & Riley, 1978). Creese has hypothesized that dopaminergic supersensitivity induced by dopamine receptor blockade by neuroleptics may be the essential pathophysiology of tardive dyskinesia. Similarly, increased dopamine receptors in schizophrenia may account for movement disorders including stereotypies.

Side effects of dopaminergic drugs have assisted in postulating the biochemical basis of OCD. Rylander (1969) reported compulsive symptoms in addicts consuming phenmetrazine. Similarly, Ellinwood (1967) reported stereotyped compulsive behavior to be an invariable component of amphetamine psychosis. Animal studies have further substantiated this finding. Ellinwood and Escalante (1970), studying cats, found compulsive movements usually consisting of repetitive sniffing of the same area continuously for 3 to 4 hours after the injection of amphetamine. Taylor and Snyder (1970) found that D-amphetamine was 10 times more potent than L-amphetamine in inducing norepinephrine-related locomotor stimulation but only twice more potent in eliciting dopamine-mediated stereotyped compulsive behavior, this implicating dopamine in the etiology of OCD. It would seem therefore that drugs that enhance dopamine level or induce dopamine receptor supersensitivity produce repetitive involuntary movements (Schildkrout, 1967).

Further supplementing the implication of dopamine in OCD is the fact that haloperidol, a dopamine receptor blocking agent has been reported to be beneficial in the treatment of Gilles de la Tourette's syndrome (Shapiro, Shapiro, & Wayne, 1973). This further supports the implication of dopamine in the production of abnormal involuntary movements. Based on these animal pharmacological and clinical findings, it has been hypothesized that OCD is the result of increased dopaminergic activity. It is worthwhile to remember that this is only a hypothesis that is far from proven. Even clinically, the tardive dyskinesia induced by neuroleptics, Huntington's chorea, or the animal pharmacological findings of stereotypies bear little resemblance to the distinctive features of OCD. If dopamine is intimately linked to OCD, it is fruitful to examine all the Parkinsonian patients treated with L-dopa for the manifestations of OCD. Even though it is a plausible hypothesis to assume that the Parkinsonian patients receiving L-dopa manifest obsessive-compulsive symptoms, many problems are raised regarding such an assumption. As these patients have bradykinesia and rigidity, many cannot perform motor rituals until such a time that their musculoskeletal system loses muscle rigidity. More important is the fact that Parkinsonian patients have low levels of dopamine in the strionigral pathways

(Barbeau, 1971). Hence, administration of L-dopa does create a dopamine excess, but in most patients, it may merely restitute to the normal level. Pharmacokinetic techniques of ascertaining plasma levels of L-dopa and correlating with the presence of obsessive symptoms pose other problems. For example, body fluid levels do not reflect the regional level in the strionigral area, and it is the level in this region that is responsible for symptom formation. Furthermore, L-dopa has been reported to modify gamma amino butric acid (Barbeau, 1971) and also decrease the pyridoxine level. It also is perplexing that Parkinsonian patients with decreased dopamine in the strionigral system suffer from depression frequently (Robins, 1976) and that OCD patients with the hypothesized hyperdopaminergic state also are vulnerable to depression. Notwithstanding these complexities, Anden (1970) reported that high doses of L-dopa produced a compulsive behavior of hammering nails into the walls in a male Parkinsonian patient. Further support for the role of dopamine in OCD awaits studies of large groups of Parkinsonian patients receiving L-dopa. Furthermore, it may well be worth employing dopamine-blocking agents in clinical treatment trials of OCD (Crawford, 1973).

Dopaminergic systems are modulated by the cholinergic (Janowski, Davis, El Yousef, & Sekerke, 1972) and serotonergic (Prange, Sisk, Wilson, Morris, Hall, & Carman, 1972) systems. In fact, for Parkinsonian patients with lower dopamine in the strionigral area, the most fruitful treatment is to give anticholinergic drugs based on the reciprocal relationship between these two extremes. Thus, Carman (1972) proposed that OCD might be treated with a dopaminolytic or a cholinomimetric or a serotonergic drug.

Thoren et al. (1980) studied the cerebrospinal fluid levels of the serotonin metabolite 5-hydroxy indoleacetic acid (5 H1AA) in OCD patients and 37 healthy controls. The mean

5 H1AA levels in the OCD patients was 123 ± 53 and $107 \pm n$ mole/L in the healthy controls. There was no significant difference in H1AA levels between the two groups. However, patients with low pretreatment H1AA level were noted to respond poorly to clomipramine (a powerful potentiator of CHS serotonin). The authors speculated the possibility of serotonin deficiency, which, on the one hand, would produce thè low pretreatment 5 H1AA in these patients and, on the other hand, would account for their poor response, for example, insufficient potentiation with clomipramine.

As a number of pure serotonergic compounds such as zimelidine are currently under investigation, they will be good investigative tools to further explore the role of serotonin biochemically and, to evaluate their efficacy clinically in the treatment of OCD. Finally, the possibility that OCD is neither a homogenous clinical syndrome nor a biochemically distinct entity should be considered. At present, one can only speculate whether these different phenomenological subtypes of OCD may represent different biochemical substrates.

PHARMACOLOGICAL TREATMENT

Neuroleptics

Garmany, May, and Folkson (1954) administered chlorpromazine to a group of five obsessive neurotic patients (two males and three females) aged between 28 and 51 years and noted that tension decreased but obsessional thinking continued unabated. Similarly, Trethowan and Scott (1955) concluded that chlorpromazine produced little relief of obsessive symptoms in 59 patients, but they noted that anxiety, tension, aggressive urges, and hypochondriacal ideas were reduced. Vidal and Vidal (1963) make references to the usefulness of methotrimeprazine as well as chlorpromazine in decreasing tension and in facilitating psychotherapeutic intervention. Altschuler (1962) treated a group of patients with obsessive rituals with 60 to 90 mg of trifluoperazine for a period of 6 months. Their schizophrenic patients did well, whereas only one of the three pure obsessionals improved.

The reported success of haloperidol in alleviating the symptoms of Gilles de la Tourette syndrome, and the observed similarity between the compulsive pattern of coprolalia and the compulsive behavior seen in OCD (Chapel, 1966; Singer, 1963; Shapiro et al., 1973) have, not surprisingly, led several investigators to try haloperidol in the treatment of OCD. O'Reagan (1970) reported that 5 mg of haloperidol daily virtually improved two OCD patients. On the other hand, Hussain and Ahad (1970) reported that haloperidol was not effective in their three patients. Thus, the available literature speaks more against than for the usefulness of neuroleptics in the treatment of obsessive disorder. However, there is no proven work to discard this group of medications either. O'Reagan's positive results supplement the statement by Shader (1970) that anxious obsessional patients with poor reality testing responded better to neuroleptics than anxiolytics. In practice, routine use of this group of drugs is definitely not indicated in OCD. Among obsessional patients, those with poor reality testing and also those who resist their symptoms minimally indicating that their symptoms may not be ego alien, are probably good candidates for haloperidol. In addition, those in whom virtually all modalities of treatment have been exhausted should also receive a trial therapy with haloperidol. It is also possible that biochemically, only those patients with the hyperdopaminergic state improve with neuroleptics. Clinically, there is no way at present to identify them.

Anxiolytics

Traditionally, anxiety has been conceptualized as the basic psychopathology in obsessive disorders. In most patients, obsessive ideas are associated with high anxiety levels that compel the individual to neutralize them by performing rituals. Can one then stop rituals simply by removing anxiety? This question, of course, has considerable theoretical impact, in addition to being a plausible therapeutic rationale.

In most patients, obsessions start very early in the teen years, followed by anxiety, and only years later depression sets in. Therefore, removal of anxiety may, in fact, prevent depression, on the one hand, and decrease obsessions, on the other hand. Theoretically, the delicate cogwheel of obsessions, anxiety, and depression poses a formidable problem of understanding the relationship between the three symptoms. Anxiolytic therapies and their response may perhaps help us understand this relationship and enhance our knowledge of OCD. The rationale for employing anxiolytic medications is that obsessive ideas and rituals are maintained because of mounting anxiety and that alleviation of anxiety may decrease the symptoms. Brietner (1960) reported that all seven of his patients improved with chlordiazepoxide in doses up to 150 mg daily. Hussain and Ahad (1970) reported successful treatment of one patient with chlordiazepoxide up to 100 mg daily. Orvin (1967) compared oxazepam with chlordiazepoxide in a double-blind, placebo-controlled crossover trial. He found that 68% of 24 patients improved on oxazepam compared to 13% on chlordiazepoxide and none on placebo.

Bethume (1964) found that a patient with a longstanding obsessional disorder obtained ''complete relief'' with diazepam. Rao (1964), in a comparative study of 16 patients, found that the 8 diazepam-treated patients improved, compared with those treated with placebo. Even in the diazepam-treated patients, compulsions remained unabated, indicating that a decrease in anxiety alone may not be useful. However, the newer benzodiazepine derivates have now been used with better therapeutic results. Burrell, Culpan, & Newton (1974) reported that 69% of 63 patients with obsessive ruminations and 72% of 32 patients with compulsive rituals improved with bromazepam. Furthermore, as their study extended for a 7-year period, the therapeutic effects were found to be lasting. In spite of widespread use and availability of many similar benzodiazepine preparations, this group of medications has not found a place in the treatment of obsessive-compulsive neurosis. However, Dally (1967) suggests that chlordiazepoxide used in combination with antidepressant drugs may be very useful.

Tricyclic Antidepressants

The use of antidepressants in OCD was initiated by the fact that obsessive personalities develop depression when they decompensate and that involutional depression is common in people with obsessional personalities. Furthermore, patients with OCD often develop severe depression. Even though some believe that OCD is a variant of affective disorder, depression often appears to be a secondary pathology. The previously mentioned statement is related to the fact that some obsessional ideas remain even after depression is completely eliminated. Antidepressants are currently used for antiobsessive action, antidepressant action, and possibly anxiolytic action. Various antidepressant agents have been tried over the years. Imipramine, being the oldest and the first antidepressant drug, has been extensively used. There are a number of studies indicating that it is a failure (Akimoto,

Nakakuki, & Machiyama, 1960; Alzheimer, 1960; Cruz & Sarro-Martin, 1959; Kramer, 1963; Matigama, Kuroiwa, & Naruse, 1959; Visitini, 1959). Others have reported mild effects (Amat Aguirre, 1966; Boucquey, 1961; Carles Egea, 1961; Michaux, Duche & Perpinoitis, 1961; Strauss, 1959); good effects (Earle & Earle, 1960; Guyotat, Marin, Dubor, & Bonhomme, 1960; Naviau, Ruyffelaere, & Lehembre, 1966); and excellent (Gattuso & Coaciuri, 1964; Geissmann & Kammerer, 1964; Vidal & Vidal, 1963) results. A case of kleptomania as a compulsive symptom has been reported to have responded well to imipramine (Dubois & Rancurel, 1967). All these studies except those of Geissmann and Kammerer (1964) and Vidal and Vidal (1963) included primary affective disorder patients with some obsessive symptoms, and, therefore, these findings are tentative and not conclusive. The two studies with OCD patients, on the other hand, did not use specific diagnostic inclusion criteria or assessment scales for evaluating changes in obsessive symptoms.

Amitriptyline compared in a double-blind study with doxepin has been found to be beneficial in the treatment of OCD (Bauer & Novak, 1969). Recently, Snyder (1980) reported substantive improvement in two patients with OCD who were resistant to all other forms of therapy. Neither of these two patients were depressed. Similarly, Hussain and Ahad (1970) reported therapeutic benefit in two cases of OCD on 300 to 400 mg of amitriptyline daily. Although the two uncontrolled and one controlled studies alluded to the efficacy of amitriptyline, in our own double-blind comparative study (Ananth, Pecknold, Van Den Steen, & Engelsmann, 1981) with 20 OCD patients, amitriptyline did not produce statistically significant improvement in 4 weeks. This may mean that 4 weeks is not enough for amitriptyline to act. Doxepin in doses of 75 to 300 mg has also been reported to be beneficial in the treatment of this syndrome (Ananth, Solyom, Solyom, & Sookman, 1975). Freed, Kerr, & Roth (1972) reported improvement of severe obsessional states with imipramine (11), amitriptyline (3), desipramine (1) and dothiepin (1). However, none remitted completely, and the improvement was achieved only on higher doses. Interestingly, these authors followed up their patients for a mean period of 4.2 years and found that 12 of the 14 patients followed had maintained marked improvement. All these findings indicated that tricyclic antidepressants do help obsessive patients. Such an effect does not seem specific to any particular antidepressant; none would completely eliminate symptoms, and in most patients a dose of 200 to 300 mg daily may be needed. These encouraging clues need to be tempered with healthy skepticism because of a number of methodological problems that will be alluded to later.

Clomipramine

Clomipramine is the only pharmacological agent that has been investigated exhaustively for treating obsessive disorders. Most of the early reports that clomipramine may be effective in OCD consisted of observations that obsessive symptoms improved in depressed patients treated with this drug. Cordoba and Lopez-Ibor Alino (1967) noted that obsessions improved in four depressed patients treated with clomipramine, oral or parenteral, up to 450 mg a day. Jimenz-Garcia (1967) reported improvement of obsessive symptoms in 3 patients with only 75 mg a day. Lopez-Ibor Alino (1969) reported that of the 16 patients treated with intravenous clomipramine up to 150 mg per day, 13 improved and 3 did not. On the other hand, Laboucarie Rascol, Jorda, Gurand, and Leinadier (1967) did not find any improvement with intravenous clomipramine or electroconvulsive therapy (ECT).

Among the anecdotal reports, 36 of the 51 patients were reported to have improved. However, these results pose important methodological problems.

First, these reports may mean that obsessional symptoms that are simply a part of depressive disease may improve because of the drug's antidepressant property, thereby reflecting that clomipramine is a good antidepressant drug. Supporting the relationship of obsession and depression, Gittelson (1966a, 1966b, 1966c, 1966d) reported that 52 of 398 depressed patients in the studies showed frank obsessional symptoms prior to the onset of symptoms. Similarly, Kendell and Discipio (1970) not only confirmed the previously mentioned findings but also noted that the obsessional symptoms correlated with the depth of depression. Secondly, what needs to be treated has to be identified and defined initially. The previously mentioned studies did not have definitive criteria for obsessive symptoms. The preoccupations of depressed patients may be mistaken for obsessive symptoms, and thus what is measured becomes doubtful. Thirdly, all of these studies did not employ any formal rating scales, and thus the improvement noted basically reflected the clinicians' judgment with associated bias. Thus, these reports did not provide definitive answers.

Uncontrolled Studies. Although anecdotal findings were reported by many, a number of studies with standardized assessments also reported improvement of obsessive symptomatology. Initial studies were designed primarily to assess the efficacy of clomipramine in the treatment of depression. Escobar, Teeter, Tuason, and Schiele (1976) found a reduction in Item 21 of the Hamilton Psychiatric Scale for depression in a 20-patient study. In our early study (Campbell, Gomez, Ananth, Bronheim, Klingner, & Ban, 1973) with 10 patients designed primarily to test the efficacy of clomipramine in the treatment of depression, a statistically significant reduction in the obsessive-compulsive cluster of the Wittenborn Scale was noted. However, improvement of obsessive symptoms in depressed patients is not valid proof of the efficacy of clomipramine against obsessions. There are a number of uncontrolled clinical trials involving the use of formal rating scales on patients with OCD. Marshall and Micev (1973) found that those obsessionals with hysterical features improved whereas those without did not. Marshall (1971), impressed with the similarity between obsessions and phobias, treated 24 phobic patients with oral clomipramine during weekends and intravenous administration during weekdays. He noted improvement in 18 patients. On further analysis, he found that 4 of the 18 patients who improved had clear-cut obsessive neurosis, and the rest were having phobic anxiety states with obsessional symptoms, which indicates that both primary and secondary obsessions improve with this drug. Although these results cannot be considered definitive as their assessment included only a 3-point scale, subsequent work (Waxman, 1973, 1975) employing a specifically developed scale based on the Leyton Obsessive Inventory indicated a 33% to 60% improvement in obsessive neurosis. Renynghe de Voxrie (1968), encouraged by spectacular results in a depressed patient with obsessive neurosis, used clomipramine in 15 refractory obsessive neurotic patients. Ten of the 15 patients were reported to have improved. Waxman (1973) treated 15 obsessive neurotic patients and a mean of 43% improvement was noted in 6 weeks. Unfortunately, they did not continue the drug for more than 6 weeks or in a dosage of more than 225 mg daily. As selection criteria for inclusion of patients into the study, assessment scales and dosage of the medication in all three studies were not definitive, we conducted a study

(Ananth *et al.*, 1979; Wyndowe, Solyom, & Ananth, 1975 in which 20 patients with a 2-year or more history of obsessive neurosis were given 75–300 mg of clomipramine with weekly assessments of obsessive-compulsive symptomatology. Self-assessments including the Social Adjustment Scale (Weissman & Bothwell, 1976), Maudsley Personality Inventory (Eysenck, 1959) and the Self Analysis Form were completed by the patients before and after the trial. Our results indicated that there was a statistically significant improvement in the severity of obsessions and anxiety by the end of 1 week and in the number of obsessive symptoms by the end of 2 weeks. Thus, a clear antiobsessive effect of clomipramine was demonstrated. However, as obsessive symptoms may spontaneously remit, all the improvement cannot be attributed to clomipramine, and thus a placebo control group is needed. Similarly, it is also important to prove the superiority of clomipramine over the existing drugs. We compared the results of two of our independent studies on OCD (Ananth & Van Den Steen, 1977), one employing doxepin (Ananth *et al.*, 1975), and the other, clomipramine (Ananth *et al.*, 1979), which revealed the superiority of clomipramine. However, as they are two independent samples, a comparison of the results is not unequivocally valid.

Placebo-Controlled Double-Blind Studies. There are a few double-blind placebo-controlled studies. Karabanow (1977) conducted a double-blind clinical trial in which 20 clinically depressed patients with obsessive-compulsive and phobic traits were randomly allocated to either a placebo or clomipramine group of equal size. The treatment consisted of 100 mg of clomipramine or an identical placebo for 6 weeks. Significant differences were noted between the placebo and the active drug group in the depression scores of the Zung Self Analysis form and on the phobia, obsessional scores of the Beaumont-Seldrup Scale. An interesting 4-month study of Yaryura-Tobias, Neziroglu, and Bergman (1976) consisted of administration of 300 mg of clomipramine daily with a placebo period of 2 weeks inserted near the middle, the time of which was double blind. Half the sample were on the placebo between 4 and 6 weeks, whereas the other half received the placebo between 6 and 8 weeks. The authors noted significant increases in ruminations during the end of the placebo period when compared with the psychopathology prior to placebo. They also noted that, in half of the patients who received the placebo at the end of 4 weeks, increase in depression scores beyond that at baseline occurred. Both these placebo-controlled studies favor clomipramine in the treatment of OCD. However, the first study included depressed patients and the second did not have a comparative placebo group.

Standard Controlled Studies. There are a number of standard drug-controlled trials. In a 4-week double-blind comparative trial (Ananth *et al.*, 1981), the therapeutic efficacy of clomipramine was compared with that of amitriptyline with weekly assessments of 20 OCD patients. Statistically significant improvement in obsessive symptoms was moted in the clomipramine group only. There was no correlation between the change in depression scores and that in obsession scores or the initial depression score and the outcome. Thoren *et al.* (1980), in a 6-week placebo-controlled study, compared the efficacy of 150 mg of clomipramine with that of nortriptyline or placebo in 24 patients randomly assigned equally into the three groups. Significant change was noted on the obsessive compulsive subscale of the Comprehensive Psychiatric Rating Scale (CPRS) that was employed for assessment in the study, whereas the depression subscale did show only a trend. However, the changes in the scores of the Leyton Obsessive Inventory were not significant. This may be related to the small number of patients included in the study.

Combination Treatments

In a multicenter study, Cassano, Castrogiovanni, and Mauri (1981) evaluated the efficacy of clomipramine alone, clomipramine with haloperidol, and clomipramine with diazepam in 64 inpatients for 60 days in a double-blind design. Nineteen patients received 25 to 250 mg of clomipramine daily, 18 received 75 to 175 mg of clomipramine with 3 to 7 mg of haloperidol daily, and 17 received 50 to 225 mg of clomipramine with 20 to 40 mg of diazepam daily. The Hamilton Rating Scale for Depression, Brief Psychiatric Rating Scale, and the Inpatient Multidimensional Psychiatric Scale were employed for assessment. The results indicated a significant reduction of psychopathology in all three groups, but the improvement was greater in the clomipramine group. Clomipramine showed a trend toward greatest and most constant improvement in obsessive-compulsive symptomatology, clomipramine and haloperidol in phobic symptomatology, as well as anxiety, tension, and excitement, and clomipramine and diazepam in insomnia. Basically, this study indicated not only the efficacy of clomipramine in the treatment of obsessive disorder but also indicated that the combinations employed were not superior to clomipramine alone. However, the sample did not fit the criteria for the diagnosis of OCD, and Cassano et al. did not have a specific rating scale for the assessment of obsessions. Regarding the result, clomipramine only produced a trend but no significant improvement on obsessive symptoms, which may be attributed to the previously mentioned problems.

Antidepressant Drugs and Behavior Therapy

Turner, Hersen, Bellack, Andrasik, and Capparell (1980) treated four patients with different treatments, thus employing the patients as their own control. The treatments included placebo, imipramine, imipramine and response prevention, and partial and total response prevention periods in four patients. The results indicated that responses were all variable in their sample. Their first patient did not respond to any treatment. During the response-prevention period, rituals decreased with a simultaneous increase in anxiety and depression ratings. In the second patient, imipramine clearly demonstrated beneficial effects that dissipated upon drug withdrawal. In the third patient, imipramine aggravated anxiety, bizarre thoughts, handwashing, and checking, and it induced auditory hallucinations. Response prevention also induced an increase in psychopathology. Although doxepin or combined doxepin and thought stopping were ineffective, combined doxepin and covert sensitization were effective. Turner *et al.* rightly point out that individual patient responses are variable, and patients respond to different treatments. However, the possibility that their second patient was a schizophrenic cannot be ruled out.

Marks, Stern, Mawson, Cobb, and McDonald (1980) developed a 40-patient study with a very complex design consisting of 4 weeks of drug or placebo and 6 weeks of additional behavioral therapy. At the end of this period, the patients were continued on a placebo or a drug again for another 26 weeks. They included only those patients who had rituals severe enough to be hospitalized. Clomipramine produced significant changes in self-rating but not in observer rating, both in mood as well as rituals. Behavioral therapy with the drug produced significantly greater improvement than the improvement in placebo-treated patients. Follow-up after 1 year indicated that the drug-treated group tended to maintain their superior improvement. As the study did not have a drug-only group, the improvement noted in the drug group may reflect either a drug-only or a drug-behavioral therapy inter-actional effect. However, retrospectively, they selected two groups of five patients each who were the most and the least depressed and then compared their changes in psychopathology during treatment. Marks *et al.* noted that the most depressed group had shown more improvement and that the least depressed changed very little. This finding indicates that the antiobsessive effect is secondary to antidepressive effect. However, the same authors noted that patients on drugs had maintained their superior improvement. If the drug is only an antidepressant, why, then, would it maintain improvement in patients after the depressive symptoms are removed? Similarly, why would they relapse to an obsessive state upon drug withdrawal? These questions need to be answered in the future. Furthermore, the authors included patients who were clinically depressed and those whose rituals were severe enough to merit hospitalization. Rachman, Cobb, Grey, McDonald, Mawson, Sartory, and Stern reported similar findings by further analysis of the same data.

This work indicates the intricate link between obsessions and depression, the unraveling of which may facilitate our understanding of obsessive psychopathology. Similarly Amin Ban, Pecknold, and Klinger (1977) assessed treatment effects in a study that included an equal number of patients (four in each group) in a clomipramine-behavioral-therapy group, a clomipramine-simulated behavioral therapy group, and a placebo behavioral therapy group for a period of 24 weeks. The patients were rated by a psychiatrist who was unaware of the treatment. Similar to the other studies, a statistically significant improvement was noted only in the combined behavioral therapy clomipramine group. On the other hand, unlike the other studies, behavioral therapy alone did not produce significant improvement. The use of a drug with simulated behavioral therapy unexpectedly fared poorly. Surprisingly, the placebo behavioral therapy group had more side effects than drug-simulated behavioral therapy indicating perhaps that the increased anxiety was reported as adverse effects. The study suffers from the problem of small sample and a lack of a specfic scale for the measurement of obsessions other than the Wittenborn Psychiatric Rating Scale. On the other hand, somewhat different from the findings of Marks *et al.* (1980) are the results of Solyom and Sookman (1977) who compared the effects of flooding (nine patients), thought stopping (eight patients), and clomipramine (six patients) in a 6-month study with a biweekly therapeutic program. They included a variety of psychiatric and psychometric measures. They noted that clomipramine had a substantial ameliorating effect on the number and severity of obsessional symptoms, reducing the severity by half. The trends suggested that the drug was as effective as flooding and more effective than thought stopping in reducing the ruminative symptoms. However, it was considerably less effective than behavioral therapy in reducing the compulsive symptoms. This indicates differential effects of drug and behavioral therapy not only on mood but also on other obsessional symptoms. Future studies should measure the effects of therapies on all the obsessional symptoms including rituals, ruminations, horrific temptations, pervading doubt, phobias, depression, and anxiety to assess both qualitative and quantitative changes.

Most studies indicate that clomipramine does not eradicate obsessive disorder. The urge to perform an act may remain, but the emotional force attached to the urge goes away. When medication is withdrawn, the symptoms may return, and the dosages necessary to improve the symptoms are in the higher range of 150 to 300 mg daily (Insel & Murphy, 1981).

Thus, all the available evidence seems to indicate that tricyclic antidepressants may have an antiobessional effect. In spite of the scarcity of patients with obsessional disorder, double-blind studies have been available to indicate such an effect. Is this effect exclusive to only clomipramine? The evidence to the contrary that other tricyclic antidepressants may have a similar effect is documented. However, clomipramine is the most potent and the most investigated. Second, the question as to whether other serotonin uptake blockers act similarly is both theoretically interesting and clinically important. Hence, a drug like zimeldine, which is a pure serotonin uptake inhibitor, should be used. Third, the relationship of antidepressive and antiobsessive effects needs to be clearly established. Marks et al. (1980) have shown elegantly the differential effects of behavioral therapy and clompiramine on mood and obsessional symptoms. The understanding of the relationship between anxiety, depression, and obsession may in itself add a new dimension to its treatment. Fourth, the evidence that behavioral and drug therapies have differential effects on ruminations as well as pervasive doubts and rituals (behavioral treatment) is clinically important even though tentative. Last, the current evidence is compelling to indicate that clomipramine is the drug of choice for OCD. It is as safe as any other first-generation antidepressant preparation available. Drug and behavioral therapy can be employed together possibly with additive or synergetic effect.

Monoamine Oxidase Inhibitors (MAOI)

Even though MAOIs have been available for a long time, there are no controlled studies of the efficacy of this group of drugs in the treatment of OCD, and MAOIs are generally considered not useful in the treatment of pure obsessional disorders (Dally, 1967). However, Annesley (1969) described a 49-year-old man with anxiety, phobias, and disabling obsessions and compulsive rituals whose symptoms gradually remitted over a 6-week period after starting phenelzine. Even after 6 months, the patient maintained improvement with 60 mg daily. Jain, Swinson, and Thomas (1970) reported a case of a 26-year-old man with anxiety, phobias, and severe disabling ruminations who lost all his symptoms over a 2-week period. Moreover, he was reported to be free of symptoms at a 4-month follow-up. Prior treatment failures in these patients included behavior therapy, ECT, insulin therapy, phenothiazines, tricyclic antidepressants, benzodiazepines, and bilateral rostral leucotomy. Another 52-year-old female patient who had lived in social isolation because of compulsive handwashing was reported to have improved on 75 mg of phenelzine daily (Isberg, 1981). The improvement is not specific to phenelzine but is related to the MAOI activity. Such an assumption is substantiated by the report of Jenike (1981) who described a 22-year-old woman and a 39-year-old man who responded rapidly to tranylcypromine therapy.

These findings assume special importance because of the following reasons. Recently, two types of MAO have been found (Youdim, 1973). MAO-A is responsible for deamination of serotonin and norepiniphrine whereas MAO-B is responsible for the deamination of benzylamine and B-phenylamine. Pure inhibitors of A (clorgyline) or B type (deprenyl) are available for investigation. These drugs may prove to be of value clinically in the future. Furthermore, in one report, a patient has been reported to have improved even though the response to imipramine was not favorable. One can then assume that there may be a MAOI responsive and a tricyclic responsive subgroup. But, unfortunately, we do not have any means of identifying them.

Lithium

The use of lithium is based on the similarity between the cyclic nature of bipolar affective disorders and the cyclic nature of some cases of OCD. In a report of a single patient, Frossman and Walinder (1969) noted a 35-year-old woman who stopped her long-standing handwashing compulsions on lithium carbonate. Van Putten and Sanders (1975) reported only partial improvement on symptoms in a 25-year-old male whose brother had a lithium-sensitive psychosis. Stern and Jenike (1982) reported remarkable improvement in a 35-year-old female patient on a serum lithium level of 0.06 to 1.0 mEq per liter. Two weeks after, lithium was discontinued, and her symptoms returned. Even though these case reports provide some evidence on the possibility of the usefulness of this substance in the treatment of obsessive disorders, controlled trials have not substantiated such a hope. Geisler and Schou (1969), in a double-blind crossover study with six obsessive-compulsive neurotic patients, found that lithium was "inactive as placebo."

Other Medications

L-tryptophan has been tried in the treatment of the obsessive disorders based on the hypothesis that an altered serotonin metabolism may be the central pathophysiology. Such a theory has received some credibility because of the promising results obtained with clomipramine. Yaryura-Tobias and Bhagawan (1977) reported improvement in five of their seven patients. In two others, pretreatment aggressive behavior increased. In another patient, headache was noted. As biochemical assessments were not included, it is not possible to attribute improvement to enhanced central serotonin.

Beta adrenergic blocking agents have been used on the hypothesis that a decrease in anxiety can be attained by decreasing the peripheral adrenergic activity. Furthermore, such an experiment is theoretically useful in that a failure of beta blockers to provide relief would assign the prime place to cognitive factors in OCD. Thus, it may help to resolve the problem of the chicken- or the egg- first situation of whether anxiety is responsible for rituals or whether rituals *per se* produce anxiety. In a 12-patient crossover study, Rabavilas, Boulougouris, Perissaki, and Stefanis (1979) noted that 300 mg daily of protalol effectively blocked the peripheral autonomic symptoms, and yet the obsessive symptoms remained unaltered. In addition, there was no improvement of subjective anxiety. Even though these findings lend support to the conclusion that the cognitive factors are crucial in the genesis of anxiety, cautious scrutiny is needed. Perhaps the short duration of drug treatment and the lack of improvement in subjective anxiety suggests the possibility of insufficient treatment.

Methyl amphetamine abreaction (Slater & Roth, 1969), narcotherapy (Kalinowsky & Hippius, 1969) with thiopentone, meprobamate (Sargant & Slater, 1950), carbon dioxide inhalations (Sargant & Slater, 1950), lysergic acid diethylamide (Dally 1967), and reserpine (Kalinowsky & Hippius, 1969) have all been tried, and such treatments are of historic interest only.

PSYCHOSURGERY

Despite the progress that has been achieved in psychiatry, there are still a certain number of patients who do not respond to treatment and who remain in great distress and nonfunctional. Such is the case with some patients with OCD. As these patients consider their symptoms ego dystonic, they are literally tormented by their symptoms. The family members also go through an agonizing time watching helplessly and trying desperately with little hope to find a miracle to improve the patient. It is these patients who are generally subjected to psychosurgery.

Psychosurgery was planned and tried first (1890) by Burckhardt at a time when no other treatment was available; it was rediscovered and reintroduced by Moniz in 1936, and it was popularized by Freeman and Watts (1944). Subsequently, because of the overuse and uncritical selection of patients, this mode of treatment has faded away. However, several highly selective neurosurgery procedures have been introduced that have revitalized interest in this mode of treatment.

The indications for psychosurgery nowadays are restricted. The main indications are intractable obsessional disorder, depression, and anxiety (Kelly, 1976). Even though there has been a proliferation of anxiolytic agents and second- and even third-generation antidepressants, and they have assessed, obsessional disorder resistance to their treatments is considered an indication for psychosurgery.

What are the side effects? A number of side effects and sequelae of psychosurgery have been reported. Although the earlier studies reported about 2% to 4% mortality (Freeman & Watts, 1944; Tooth & Newton, 1961), later studies with new techniques of stereotactic procedures have eliminated operative mortality (Post, Rees, & Schurr, 1968; Sykes & Tredgold, 1964). The second serious change is epilepsy which occurred in 16% after restricted operation of orbital undercutting. Stereotactic tractotomy is virtually devoid of this side effect (1 in 210 patients). Personality changes following psychosurgery (postleucotomy syndrome) was a sequel to standard leucotomy. With much restricted, open, or stereotactic procedures, undesirable personality changes are minimal. Hence, side effects or sequelae should not be deterrents for the use of psychosurgery in needy patients.

What is the rationale for the operation? Both anatomic and physiological studies have shown that the limbic lobe is related to emotion. Cingulate projections (Nauta, 1964) and pathways from the orbital cortex to uncus (Van Hoesen, Pandya, & Butters, 1972) appear to be important in psychiatric disorders characterized by stereotypy of an excessive and futile response including anxiety, phobia, and obsessions. Lewin (1973) confirmed the relatively specific associations linking affective disturbances with the orbital regions and obsessional symptoms with cingulate gyrus. In mixed states, he noted the disappearance of depression following orbital lesions and obsessions following cingulate lesions. Meyer, McElhaney, Martin, and McGraw (1973) also noted that both obsessional and depressive patients did well with cingulectomies. However, at present there is no neurophysiological evidence to support specific neuronal pathways mediating obsessive behavior. At this point, these operations are based on empirical evidence only.

Is it a cure or temporary relief of symptoms? Most psychiatric therapy only affects the symptoms temporarily, and in some cases (schizophrenia), medication needs to be continued for a long time to prevent relapses. Even lithium, which is considered a prophylactic, needs to be continued to prevent recurrences. If psychosurgery improves symptoms, is it then a curative treatment? Many of the follow-up studies indicate lasting relief. However, we followed a young male obsessive who had excellent relief of symptoms for an approximately 2- to 3-year period that was followed by a recurrence. He underwent psychosurgery three times. He is now suffering from obsessive symptoms again. At this point, it is hard to answer the question whether psychosurgery is curative or whether the effect dissipates over time. Studies that depict the clinical state of each patient over time are needed. Generally favorable response in patients with obsessive symptoms was noted by Sargent (1962), Holden, Itil, and Hofstatter (1970) and Pippard (1955). On the other hand, Bonis, Covello, and Lemperiere (1968) reported that a patient with obsessional neurosis not only failed to respond but developed new symptoms of impulsivity and irritability. However, the problems with psychosurgery lie in the limited accurately localized lesions that are sufficient enough to produce the desired clinical effect but without any untoward effects, including personality change and organic brain syndrome. The correlation of these lesions with their clinical and neuropathological effects will be both interesting and rewarding. The recent advances have made such limited lesions possible, and therefore many limited operations have been tried to improve OCD.

Orbital Undercutting

Knight (1969) and Scoville (1960) commented that obsessives did not change with psychosurgery. On the other hand, Sykes and Tredgold (1964), primarily focusing their attention on obsessive patients, noted improvement in tension and scrupulousness after orbital undercutting. Everyone showed benefit for some time, but only 50% maintained significant improvement. Even though the obsessional symptoms persisted, they were less disabling. In spite of this improvement, the capacity for leisure-time enjoyment was decreased. In addition, there was a mortality rate of 1.5%, convulsions in 12%, and personality change in 16%.

Stereotactic Tractotomy

Bridges, Goktepe, Maratos, Browne, and Young (1973) treated 24 obsessional patients by means of a bilateral stereotactic tractotomy with assessments similar to the previously mentioned study. Sixteen patients improved well, 6 improved mildly, and 2 did not change in a 3-year follow-up. Strom-Olsen and Carlisle (1971) reported on 210 patients of which 150 were available for follow-up with relatives 16 months to 8 years after surgery. They noted complete recovery in 33% and "much improvement" in another 16%. They reported an improvement rate of 40% in obsessives.

Anterior Cingulectomy

From Sydney, Australia, Hohne and Walsh (1970) reported on the results of anterior cingulectomy in 48 depressed patients. The surgery was conducted under direct vision. Among the 48 patients operated were 7 each anxiety, phobic, depressive, and obsessive-compulsive sufferers. Full remission along with restoration of ability to function at a prepsychotic level was noted in 88% of the patients. The authors commented on "the life-saving usefulness" of this type of surgery.

Bimedial Leucotomy

In the first study, Marks, Birley, and Gelder (1966) matched 22 disabled, phobic neurotic patients operated on between 1952 and 1962 with 16 suitable controls. The operations were bimedial leucotomies in the coronal plane just anterior to ventricular horn. Blind raters noted that the leucotomy patients did significantly better than controls with respect to phobias and general anxiety. Tan, Marks, and Marset (1971) also restrospectively analyzed 24 obsessive-compulsive neurotic patients who had had a leucotomy (bimedial operation) and 13 matched controls (Post et al., 1968). Comparison 5 years after treatment indicated that the leucotomy group did significantly better than controls with respect to obsessions and generalized anxiety. Their obsessions were not cured but were reduced from a severe to a moderate degree with only a mild personality change. Shobe and Gildea (1968) reported a 6- to 18-year follow-up study of patients who had medical leucotomy in the nondominant hemisphere only. Most patients selected were "obsessive-compulsive, phobic, hypochondriacal, or tense and anxious in addition to having depression with agitation. Excellent improvement was noted in 18 of the 22 patients that persisted for 6 to 18 years. In the Lahey Clinic, follow-up of 8 to 22 years duration (Tucker, 1966) reported good results after bimedial open leucotomy in 14 of the 20 OCD patients. Baker, Young, and Gould (1970) noted that OCD patients with phobic symptoms responded better than "classic obsessive-compulsive neurotic patients."

In a follow-up of 43 private psychiatric patients (Bernstein, Callahan, & Jaranson 1975) referred for open bimedial prefrontal lobotomies between 1948 and 1970, patients were evaluated by clinical interviews and review of medical records for assessing improvement, emergence of the organic brain syndrome, and side effects. Twenty-seven of the 43 patients included in the follow-up were obsessive-compulsive neurotic patients, all of whom had severe impairment not amenable to treatment. All improved to a varying degree. Twelve patients had mild (11) to moderate (2) organic brain syndrome. Five patients developed postoperative seizures, and 10 developed obesity.

Limbic Leucotomy

Kelly, Walter, and Mitchell-Heggs (1972) followed obsessive neurotic patients with regular assessment prior to and after pyschosurgery. The extensive assessment included the Taylor Manifest Anxiety Scale, the Maudsley Personality Inventory, the Beck Depression Scale, and the Leyton Obsessional Inventory. There was an 80% therapeutic response. All these patients had a cingulate and lower medial quadrant operations (limbic leucotomy). On the Leyton Obsessive Inventory, there was significant reduction in obsessional symptoms, in the degree of resistance to the obsessional symptoms, and in the interference by the obsessions ($p < .001$).

Now, what is the place of psychosurgery in the modern era? A number of factors have to be considered carefully. The factors associated with favorable prognosis are good premorbid personality, stable home environment, good work record, late onset, short duration, presence of anxiety and tension, and absence of long-standing rituals (Linford-Rees, 1973; Sykes & Tredgold, 1964). However, these are the very patients who improve with other forms of therapies as well. Environmental factors necessary for a good prognosis include well-planned postoperative care and rehabilitation. A supportive family or institutional milieu is necessary during the postoperative phase.

All the available evidence indicates that psychosurgery may have a place for a number of the unfortunate victims of obsessions and ruminations who continue to be tortured in spite of all treatment. Miller (1972) has summarized the place of psychosurgery as follows:

Psychosurgery is no panacea, but is sometimes a godsend in serious and disabling mental illness. Its results are unpredictable, but in selected cases, they may be exceptionally good, and there can be no doubt whatever that when it is carried out after mature and considered judgment and by skilled hands, its

benefits far outweigh its hazards—psychosurgery is certainly not
a subject for denounciation or prohibition, but needs the cool,
continuous scientific consideration that should be applied to all
problematical forms of treatment. (p. 190)

Most concur with Miller that this valuable treatment should
not have a sad demise, but, at the same time, it should only
be used as a last recourse.

CONCLUSION

Obsessive disorders form a distinct psychiatric syndrome
that is easy to diagnose and difficult to treat. Many authors
in the past have indicated a grave prognosis for this disorder
(Templer, 1972). Pollitt (1957) has pointed out that "true obsessional states are among the few illnesses that can still torture patients almost for a lifetime." Such a prognosis was perhaps justified in the past, but it does not apply for the current
time because tremendous progress has been made in pharmacological, psychosurgical, as well as behavioral therapies.

In the pharmacotherapy of OCD, antidepressants are particularly promising. Even though all antidepressants may be
useful in varying degrees, two facts must be borne in mind.
First, the response of a particular patient to a drug is unpredictable. Second, of the various antidepressants, clomipramine
is the most extensively investigated and the most promising
in the treatment of OCD. There are indications that it may
have specific antiobsessive effects. Even though predictive indices are not available, patients with depressive symptomatology and ruminators have been reported to respond well. Finally, when used, doses of up to 300 mg daily should be tried
before concluding that the patient is nonresponsive. Relapses
are to be expected upon withdrawal of the drug, and be-

havioral therapy, if necessary, can be added to the drug regimen with benefit.

Among the various drugs, the physician would choose the appropriate drug for a particular patient, depending on the predominant psychopathology, past treatment results, and the availability of drugs. Depending on the psychopathological profile at the time of presentation, an anxiolytic to relieve the coexisting anxiety and antidepressants to relieve the predominant depressive symptoms are desirable. Perhaps, neuroleptics can be used with a maximum therapeutic advantage in those obsessive patients with associated psychotic symptoms.

REFERENCES

Akimoto, H., Nakakuki, M., & Machiyama, Y. Clinical experiences with MAO inhibitors (a comparison with Tofranil). *Diseases of the Nervous System*, 1960, *21*, 645–647.

Altschuler, M. Massive doses of trifluoperazine in the treatment of compulsive rituals. *American Journal of Psychiatry*, 1962, *119*, 367–368.

Alzheimer, O. Zur Pharmacotherapie depressiver erkrankungen. *Medizinische Welt*, 1960, *37*, 1918–1926.

Amat Aguirre, E. Tratamiento de las depresiones atípicas. *Revue Informacion Medicale-Therapie*, 1966, *41*, 387–392.

American Psychiatric Association. *Diagnostic and statistical manual of mental disorders* (3rd ed.). Washington, DC: Author, 1980.

Amin, M. M., Ban, T. A., Pecknold, J. C., & Klingner, A. Clomipramine (Anafranil) and behavior therapy in obsessive-compulsive and phobic disorders. *Journal of International Medical Research*, 1977, *5*, (Suppl. 5), 33–37.

Ananth, J. Pathophysiology of tardive dyskinesia. *Neuropsychobiology*, 1982, *8*, 210–212.

Ananth, J., & Van Den Steen, N. Systematic studies in the treatment of obsessive-compulsive neurosis with tricyclic antidepressants. *Current Therapeutic Research*, 1977, *21*, 495–501.

Ananth, J., Solyom, L., Solyom, C., & Sookman, D. Doxepin in the treatment of obsessive compulsive neurosis. *Psychosomatics*, 1975, *16*, 185–187.

Ananth, J., Solyom, L., Bryntwick, S., & Krishnappa, U. Clomipramine therapy for obsessive compulsive neurosis. *American Journal of Psychiatry*, 1979, *135*, 700–701.

Ananth, J., Pecknold, J., Van Den Steen, N., & Engelsmann, F. Double-blind comparative study of clomipramine and amitriptyline in obsessive neurosis. *Progress in Neuro-Psychopharmacology*, 1981, 5, 257–262.

Anden, N. G. Oral L-dopa treatment of Parkinsonism. *Acta Medica Scandinavica*, 1970, 187, 247–255.

Annesley, P. T. Nardil response in a chronic obsessive compulsive. *British Journal of Psychiatry*, 1969, 115, 748.

Baker, E. F. W., Young, M. P., & Gould, D. M. A new look at bimedial prefrontal leukotomy. *Canadian Medical Association Journal*, 1970, 102, 37–41.

Barbeau, A. Long-term side effects of levodopa. *Lancet*, 1971, 1, 395.

Bauer, G., & Novak, H. Doxepine ein neuves Antidepressivum; Wirkungvergleich mit Amitriptylin. *Arzneimittel-Forschung*, 1969, 19, 1642–1646.

Bernstein, I., Callahan, W. A., & Jaranson, J. M. Lobotomy in private practice. *Archives of General Psychiatry*, 1975, 32, 1041–1047.

Bethume, H. C. A new compound in the treatment of anxiety states: Report on the use of diazepam. *New Zealand Medical Journal*, 1964, 63, 153–156.

Black, A. The natural history of obsessional neurosis. In H. H. Beech, H. H. (Ed.), *Obsessive states*. London: Methuen, 1974.

Bonis, A., Covello, L., & Lemperiere, T. Etude critique des indications d' interventions psychochirurgicales. *Encephale*, 1968, 57, 439–473, 525–563.

Boucquey, J., & Boucquey, J. P. Traitement ambulatoire à l'imipramine de 50 cas de psychoneurosis. *Revue Médicale de Louvain*, 1961, 5, 126–142.

Brickner, R. M., Rosen, A. A., & Munro, R. Physiological aspects of the obsessive state. *Psychosomatic Medicine*, 1940, 2, 369–383.

Bridges, P. K., Goktepe, E. O., Maratos, J., Browne, A., & Young, L. A comparative review of patients with obsessional neurosis and with depression treated by psychosurgery. *British Journal of Psychiatry*, 1973, 123, 663–674.

Brietner, C. Drug therapy in obsessional states and other psychiatric problems. *Diseases of the Nervous System* (Suppl.) 1960, 21, 31–35.

Brown, F. W. Heredity in psychoneuroses. *Proceedings of the Royal Society of Medicine*, 1942, 35, 785–790.

Burckhardt, G. Uber Rindenexcisionen, als Beitrag zur operativen Therapie der Psychosen. *Allgemeine Zeitschrift feur Psychiatrie*, 1890, 74, 463.

Burrell, R. H., Culpan, R. H., Newton, K. J. Use of bromazepam in obsessional, phobic and related states. *Current Medical Research Opinion*, 1974, 2, 430–436.

Campbell, B., Gomez, L., Ananth, J. V., Bronheim, L. A., Klingner, A., & Ban, T. A. An uncontrolled clinical trial with clomipramine in the treatment of depressed patients. *Current Therapeutic Research*, 1973, 15, 223–231.

Carles Egea, F. Observaciones sobre el tratamiento ambulatorio de los estados depresivos con G 22355 (Tofranil). *Medicina Clínica* (Barcelona), 1961, 36, 448–452.

Carman, J. S. Hyperdopaminergic states: A continuum. *Lancet*, 1972, *2*, 1249.

Cassano, G. G., Castrogiovanni, P., & Mauri, M. A multicenter controlled trial in phobic-obsessive psychoneurosis. The effect of chlorimipramine and its combinations with haloperidol and diazepam. *Progress in Neuropsychopharmacology*, 1981, *5*, 129–138.

Chapel, J. L. Gilles de la Tourette's disease—The past and the present. *Canadian Psychiatric Association Journal*, 1966, *11*, 324–329.

Cooper, J. E. The Leyton Obsessive Inventory. *Psychological Medicine*, 1970, *1*, 48–64.

Cordoba, E. F., & Lopez-Ibor Alino, J. J. La monochlorimiprame en enfornes psychiatrices resistantes en otros tratamientos. *Acta Luso Español Neurologi Psychiatri*, 1967, *26*, 119–147.

Crawford, J. F. Cerebral autonomic imbalance. *Lancet*, 1973, *2*, 772–773.

Creese, I., Bivet, D. R., & Snyder, S. H. Dopamine receptor binding enhancement accompanies lesion-induced behavioral supersensitivity. *Science*, 1977, *197*, 596–598.

Cruz, M. de la, & Sarro-Martin, A. Experiencias con un nuevo antidepressivo derivado del iminodibencilo. *Medicina Clínica* (Barcelona), 1959, *33*, 122–125.

Dally, P. *Chemotherapy of psychiatric disorders*. London: Logos Press, 1967.

Dubois, J. C., & Rancurel, G. Vol et melancolie: A propos de cinq observations. *Annales Médico-Psychologiques* (Paris), 1967, *125*, 572–579.

Earle, B. V., & Earle, A. M. Imipramine (Tofranil) in mental health clinic and private practice. *Canadian Medical Association Journal*, 1960, *83*, 804–806.

Ellinwood, E. H., Jr. Amphetamine psychosis. I. Description of the individuals and the process. *Journal of Nervous and Mental Disease*, 1967, *144*, 273–283.

Ellinwood, E. H., Jr., & Escalante, O. Chronic amphetamine effect on the olfactory forebrain. *Biological Psychiatry*, 1970, *2*, 189–203.

Escobar, J., Teeter, R. R., Tuason, V. B., & Schiele, B. C. Intravenous chlorimipramine and depressive subtypes. *Diseases of the Nervous System*, 1976, *37*, 325–328.

Eysenck, H. *The manual of Maudsley Personality Inventory*. London: University of London Press, 1959.

Freed, A., Kerr, T. A., & Roth, M. The treatment of obsessional neurosis. *British Journal of Psychiatry*, 1972, *120*, 590–591.

Freeman, W., & Watts, J. W. Psychosurgery: An evaluation of 200 cases over seven years. *Journal of Mental Science*, 1944, *90*, 379–532.

Frossman, H., & Walinder, J. Lithium treatment on atypical indication. *Acta Psychiatrica Scandinavica*, 1969 (Suppl. 207), 34–40.

Garmany, G., May, A. R., & Folkson, A. The use and action of chlorpromazine in psychoneuroses. *British Medical Journal*, 1954, *3*, 439–441.

Gattuso, S., & Coaciuri, V. L'imipramine nella terapia della nevrosi assessiva. *Acta Neurologica* (Napoli) 1964, *19*, 424–431.

Geisler, A., & Schou, M. Lithium for obsessive neurosis. *Nordisk Psykiatrisk Tidsskrift*, 1969, *23*, 493–495.

Geissmann, P., & Kammerer, T. L'imipramine dans la nevrose obsessionnelle. Etude de 30 cas. *Encephale*, 1964, *53*, 369–382.

Gittelson, N. L. The effect of obsessions in depressive psychosis. *British Journal of Psychiatry*, 1966, *112*, 253–259. (a)

Gittelson, N. L. The phenomenology of obsessions in depressive psychosis. *British Journal of Psychiatry*, 1966, *112*, 261–264. (b)

Gittelson, N. L. The fate obsessions in depressive psychosis. *British Journal of Psychiatry*, 1966, *112*, 705–708. (c)

Gittelson, N. L. Depressive psychosis in obsessional neurotics. *British Journal of Psychiatry*, 1966, *112*, 883–887. (d)

Goodwin, D. W., Guze, S. B., & Robins, E. Follow up studies in obsessional neurosis. *Archives of General Psychiatry*, 1969, *20*, 182–187.

Grimshaw, L. The outcome of obsessional disorder: A follow up study of 100 cases. *British Journal of Psychiatry*, 1965, *111*, 1051–1056.

Guyotat, J., Marin, A., Dubor, P., & Bonhomme, R. L'imipramine en dehors des états dépressifs. *Journal Médicale Lyon*, 1960, *41*, 367–375.

Hohne, H. H., & Walsh, K. W. *Surgical modification of personality: Mental health research project.* Melbourne, Australia: Victorian Mental Health Authority, 1970.

Holden, J. M. C., Itil, T. M., & Hofstatter, L. Prefrontal lobotomy: Stepping stone or pitfall? *American Journal of Psychiatry*, 1970, *127*, 591–598.

Hussain, M. Z., & Ahad, A. Treatment of obsessive compulsive neurosis. *Canadian Medical Association Journal*, 1970, *103*, 648–650.

Insel, T. R., & Murphy, D. L. The pharmacological treatment of obsessive-compulsive disorder: A review. *Journal of Clinical Psychopharmacology*, 1981, *1*, 304–311.

Isberg, R. S. A comparison of phenelzine and imipramine in an obsessive-compulsive patient. *American Journal of Psychiatry*, 1981, *138*, 1250–1251.

Jain, V. K., Swinson, R. P., & Thomas, J. G. Phenelzine in obsessional neurosis. *British Journal of Psychiatry*, 1970, *117*, 237–238.

Janowski, D. S., Davis, J. M., El Yousef, M. K., & Sekerke, H. J. A cholinergic adrenergic hypothesis of mania and depression. *Lancet*, 1972, *2*, 632–635.

Jenike, M. A. Rapid response of severe obsessive compulsive disorder to tranylcypromine. *American Journal of Psychiatry*, 1981, *138*, 1249–1251.

Jimenz Garcia, P. Experiencia clínica con clomipramina en enfermos psychiátricos. *Libro de Becas Cursos*, 1967, *58*, 179–201.

Kalinowsky, L. B., & Hippius, H. *Pharmacological, convulsive, and other somatic treatments in psychiatry.* New York: Grune & Stratton, 1969.

Kalinowsky, L. G., & Hoch, P. H. *Somatic treatments in psychiatry.* New York: Grune & Stratton, 1961.

Kanner, L. *Clinical psychiatry* (3rd ed.). Springfield, IL: Charles C Thomas, 1957.

Karabanow, O. Double-blind controlled study in phobias and obsessions complicated by depression. *International Journal of Medical Research*, 1977, 5, (Suppl. 5), 42-48.

Kelly, D., Walter, C. J. S., & Mitchell-Heggs, N. Modified leucotomy assessed clinically, physiologically and psychologically at six weeks and eighteen months. *British Journal of Psychiatry*, 1972, 120, 19-29.

Kelly, D. Therapeutic outcome in limbic leucotomy in psychiatric patients. *Psychiatry, Neurology, Neurosurgery* (Amsterdam), 1976, 76, 353-363.

Kendell, R. E., & Discipio, W. J. Obsessive symptoms and obsessional personality traits in patients with depressive illnesses. *Psychological Medicine*, 1970, 1, 65-72.

Klawan, H. L. The pharmacology of tardive dyskinesia. *American Journal of Psychiatry*, 1973, 130, 82-86.

Knight, G. Bifrontal stereotractotomy. *British Journal of Psychiatry*, 1969, 115, 257-266.

Kolb, L. C. *Noyse's modern clinical psychiatry*. Philadelphia: W. B. Saunders, 1968.

Kramer, M. Delirium as a complication of imipramine therapy in the aged. *American Journal of Psychiatry*, 1963, 120, 502-503.

Kringlen, E. Natural history of obsessional neurosis. *Seminars in Psychiatry*, 1970, 2, 403-419.

Laboucarie, J., Rascol, A., Jorda, P., Guraud, R., & Leinadier, H. New prospects in the treatment of melancholic states. Therapeutic study of a major antidepressant, chlorimipramine. *Revue Médicale de Toulouse*, 1967, 3, 863-872.

Lewin, W. Selective leucotomy: A review. In L. Laininen & K. E. Livingston (Eds.), *Surgical approaches in psychiatry*. England: Medical and Technical Publishing Co., Ltd., 1973.

Lewis, A. Problems of obsessional illness. *Proceedings of the Royal Society of Medicine*, 1935, 29, 325-336.

Linford-Rees, W. The value and limitations of psychosurgery in the treatment of psychiatric illness. *Psychiatry, Neurology, Neurosurgery* (Amsterdam), 1973, 76, 323-334.

Lo, W. H. A follow-up study of obsessional neurotics in Hong Kong Chinese. *British Journal of Psychiatry*, 1967, 113, 823-832.

Lopez-Ibor, Alino, J. J. Intravenous perfusion of monochlorimipramine. Techniques and results. In *Proceedings of the International College of CINP, Teragone, April, 1968 (International Congress Series, 180, 519)*. Netherlands. *Excerpta Medica*, 1969.

Marks, I. M., Birley, J. L. T., & Gelder, M. G. Modified leucotomy in severe agoraphobia: A controlled serial enquiry. *British Journal of Psychiatry*, 1966, *112*, 757–769.

Marks, I. M., Stern, R. S., Mawson, D., Cobb, J., & McDonald, R. Clomipramine and exposure for obsessive-compulsive rituals. *British Journal of Psychiatry*, 1980, *136*, 1–25.

Marshall, W. K. Treatment of obsessional illness and phobic anxiety state with clomipramine. *British Journal of Psychiatry*, 1971, *119*, 467–468.

Marshall, W. K. & Micev, V. Clomipramine in the treatment of obsessional illness and phobic anxiety states. *Journal of International Medical Research*, 1973, *1*, 403–412.

Matigama, Y., Kuroiwa, S., & Naruse, H. Some clinical experience with a new iminodibenzyl derivative G.22344 (Tofranil) (Japan). *Bulletin of the Seishin-Igaku Institute* [Clinical Psychiatry], 1959, *1*, 581–585.

Meyer, G., McElhaney, M., Martin, W., & McGraw, C. P. Stereotactic cingulotomy with results of acute stimulation and serial psychological testing. In L. Laininen & K. E. Livingston (Eds.), *Surgical Approaches in Psychiatry*. Baltimore: Baltimore University Press, 1973.

Meyer-Gross, W., Slater, E., & Roth, M. *Clinical Psychiatry*. London: Bailliere, Tindal & Cassell, 1969.

Michaux, L., Duche, D., & Perpinoitis. Etude pharmocodynamique, clinique et therapeutique du G22344 en pedo-psychiatrie. *Proceedings of the 3rd World Congress of Psychiatry, Montreal*, 1961, *2*, 927–929 (McGill, Montreal, 1961).

Miller, H. Psychosurgery & Dr. Breggin. *New Scientist*, 1972, *55*, 188–190.

Moniz, E. *Tentative opératoires dans le traitement de certaine psychoses*. Paris: Masson, 1936.

Naviau, J., Ruyffelaere, J., & Lehembre, C. A propos de deux cas de nevrose obsessionnelle. *Annales Médico-Psychologiques* (Paris) 1966, *124*, 254–258.

Nauta, W. J. H. Some efferent connections of the prefrontal cortex in the monkey. In J. W. Warren & K. Akert (Eds.), *Frontal granular cortex and behavior*. New York: McGraw-Hill, 1964.

O'Reagan, J. B. Treatment of obsessive compulsive neurosis with haloperidol. *Canadian Medical Association Journal*, 1970, *103*, 167–168.

Orvin, G. H. The treatment of the phobic obsessive compulsive patient with oxazepam, an improved benzodiazepine compound. *Psychosomatics*, 1967, *8*, 278–280.

Owen, F., Crow, T. J., Foulter, M., Cross, A. J., Longden, A., & Riley, G. J. Increased dopamine-receptor sensitivity in schizophrenia. *Lancet*, 1978, *2*, 223–226.

Philpott, R. Recent advances in the behavioral measurement of obsessional difficulties common to these and other measures. *Scottish Medical Journal*, 1975, *20*, 33–40.

Pippard, J. Rostral leucotomy: A report on 240 cases personally followed up after 1½ to 5 years. *Journal of Mental Science*, 1955, *101*, 756–773.

Pollitt, J. Natural history of obsessional states. *British Medical Journal*, 1957, *1*, 194–198.

Post, F., Rees, W. L., & Schurr, P. H. An evaluation of bimedial leucotomy. *British Journal of Psychiatry*, 1968, *114*, 1223–1246.

Prange, A. J., Sisk, J. L., Wilson, I. C., Morris, C. E., Hall, C. D., Carman, J. S. Proceedings of N.I.M.H. Serotonin Conference, Palo Alto, California. Washington: U.S. Government Printing Office, 1972.

Rabavilas, A. D., Boulougouris, J. C., Perissaki, C., & Stefanis, C. The effect of peripheral beta-blockade on psychophysiologic responses in obsessional neurotics. *Comprehensive Psychiatry*, 1979, *20*, 378–383.

Rachman, S., Cobb, J., Grey, S., McDonald, B., Mawson, D., Sartory, G., & Stern, R. The behavioral treatment of obsessive-compulsive disorders with or without clomipramine. *Behavioral Research & Therapy*, 1979, *17*, 467–478.

Rachman, S. J., & Hodgson, R. J. *Obsessions and compulsions*. Englewood Cliffs, NJ: Prentice-Hall, 1980.

Rao, A. V. A controlled trial with "valium" in obsessive compulsive state. *Journal of the Indian Medical Association*, 1964, *42*, 564–567.

Rapoport, J., Elkins, R., & Müielsen, E. A clinical controlled trial of chlorimipramine in adolescents with obsessive compulsive disorder. *Psychopharmacology Bulletin*, 1980, *16*, 61–63.

Renynghe de Voxrie, G. V. L'Anafranil dans l'obsession. *Acta Neurologica Belgica*, 1968, *68*, 787–792.

Robins, A. H. Depression in patients with Parkinsonism. *British Journal of Psychiatry*, 1976, *128*, 141–145.

Rosenberg, C. M. Complications of obsessional neurosis. *British Journal of Psychiatry*, 1968, *114*, 477–478.

Rylander, G. Clinical and medico criminological aspects of addictions to central stimulating drugs. In E. Sjoquist & E. Tottie (Eds.) *Abuse of central stimulants*. New York: Raven Press, 1969.

Sakai, T. Clinicogenetic study on obsessive compulsive neurosis. *Bulletin of Osaka Medical School*, 1968, (Suppl. 12), 323–331.

Sargant, W. & Slater, E. Discussion on the treatment of obsessional neuroses. *Proceedings of the Royal Society of Medicine*, 1950, *43*, 1007–1010.

Sargent, W. The present indications for leucotomy. *Lancet*, 1962, *1*, 1197–1200.

Schilder, P. The organic background of obsessions and compulsions. *American Journal of Psychiatry*, 1938, *94*, 1397–1416.

Schildkrout, J. J., & Kety, S. S. Biogenic amines and emotion. *Science*, 1967, *156*, 21–30.

Scoville, W. B. Late results of orbital undercutting. Report of 76 patients un-dergoing quantitative selective lobotomies. *American Journal of Psychiatry,* 1960, *117,* 525–532.

Shader, R. I. Antianxiety agents: A clinical perspective. In A. DiMascio & R. Shader (Eds.), *Clinical handbook of psychopharmacology.* New York: Science Press, 1970. 71–77.

Shapiro, A. K., Shapiro, G., & Wayne, H. Treatment of Tourette's syndrome. *Archives of General Psychiatry,* 1973, *28,* 92–97.

Shobe, F. O., & Gildea, M. C. L. Long-term follow-up of selected lobotomized private patients. *Journal of American Medical Association,* 1968, *206,* 327–332.

Singer, K. Gilles de la Tourette's disease. *American Journal of Psychiatry,* 1963, *20,* 80–81.

Slater, E., & Roth, M. *Clinical psychiatry* (3rd ed.). Baltimore, MD: William & Wilkins, 1969.

Snyder, S. Amitriptyline treatment of obsessive compulsive neurosis. *Journal of Clinical Psychiatry,* 1980, *41,* 286–289.

Solyom, L., & Sookman, D. A comparison of clomipramine hydrochloride (Anafranil) and behavioral therapy in the treatment of obsessive neurosis. *Journal of International Medical Research,* 1977, *5* (Suppl. 5), 49–61.

Stern, T. A., & Jenike, M. A. Treatment of obsessive compulsive disorder with lithium carbonate. *Psychosomatics,* 1983, *24,* 671–673.

Strauss, H. Office treatment of depressive states with a new drug (imipramine). *New York State Journal of Medicine,* 1959, *59,* 2906–2910.

Strom-Olsen, R., & Carlisle, S. Bifrontal stereotractotomy: A follow up study of its effects on 210 patients. *British Journal of Psychiatry,* 1971, *118,* 141–154.

Sykes, M. K., & Tredgold, R. F. Restricted orbital undercutting: A study of its effects on 350 patients over the ten years, 1951–1960. *British Journal of Psychiatry,* 1964, *110,* 609–640.

Tan, E., Marks, I. M., & Marset, P. Bimedial leucotomy in obsessive compulsive neurosis: A controlled serial enquiry. *British Journal of Psychiatry,* 1971, *118,* 155–164.

Taylor, K. M., & Snyder, S. H. Amphetamine differentiation of D- and L-isomers of animal behavior involving central norepinephrine or dopamine. *Science,* 1970, *168,* 1487–1489.

Templer, D. I. The obsessional neurosis: A review of research findings. *Comprehensive Psychiatry,* 1972, *13,* 375–383.

Thoren, P., Asberg, M., Cronholm, B., Jorenstedt, L., & Traskman, L. Clomipramine treatment of obsessive-compulsive disorder: A controlled clinical trial. *Archives of General Psychiatry,* 1980, *37,* 1281–1289.

Tooth, G. C., & Newton, M. P. *Leucotomy in England and Wales.* London: Her Majesty's Stationery Office, 1961.

Trethowan, W. F., & Scott, P. A. L. Chlorpromazine in obsessive-compulsive neurosis and allied disorders. *Lancet,* 1955, *1,* 781–785.

Tucker, W. I. Indications for modified leucotomy. *Lahey Clinic Foundation Bulletin*, 1966, *15*, 131–139.

Turner, S. M., Hersen, M., Bellack, A. S., Andrasik, F., & Capparell, H. V. Behavioral and pharmacological treatment of obsessive-compulsive disorders. *Journal of Nervous and Mental Disease*, 1980, *168*, 651–657.

Vanggard, T. The concept of neurosis. *Acta Psychiatrica Scandinavica*, 1959, *16*, 117–136.

Van Hoesen, G. W., Pandya, D. N., & Butters, N. Cortical afferents to the entorhinal cortex of the rhesus monkey. *Science*, 1972, *175*, 1471–1473.

Van Putten, T., & Sanders, D. G. Lithium in treatment failures. *Journal of Nervous and Mental Disease*, 1975, *161*, 255–264.

Vidal, G., & Vidal, B. Imipramine et obsessions. *Encephale*, 1963, *52*, 167–180.

Visitini, F. Terapia degli stati depressivi con Tofranil. *Giornale Psychiatrico Neuropatologico*, 1959, *30*, 3–8.

Waxman, D. A general practice investigation on the use of clomipramine in obsessional and phobic disorders. *Journal of International Medical Research*, 1973, *1*, 417–420.

Waxman, D. An investigation into the use of anafranil in phobic and obsessional disorders. *Scottish Medical Journal*, 1975, *20*, 61–66.

Weissman, M., & Bothwell, S. Assessment of social adjustment by patient self-report. *Archives of General Psychiatry*, 1976, *33*, 111–115.

Woodruff, R., & Pitts, F. M. Monozygotic twins with obsessional illness. *American Journal of Psychiatry*, 1964, *120*, 1075–1080.

Wyndowe, J., Solyom, L., & Ananth, J. Anafranil in obsessive compulsive neurosis. *Current Therapeutic Research*, 1975, *18*, 611–617.

Yaryura-Tobias, J. A., & Bhagawan, H. N. L-tryptophan in obsessive-compulsive disorders. *American Journal of Psychiatry*, 1977, *134*, 1298–1299.

Yaryura-Tobias, J. A., Neziroglu, F., & Bergman, L. Clomipramine for obsessive compulsive neurosis: An organic approach. *Current Therapeutic Research*, 1976, *20*, 541–547.

Youdim, M. B. H. Multiple forms of mitrochondrial monoamine oxidase. *British Medical Bulletin*, 1973, *29*, 120–122.

6

Future Directions in the Assessment and Treatment of Obsessive-Compulsive Disorder

MATIG MAVISSAKALIAN, SAMUEL TURNER, AND LARRY MICHELSON

The preceding chapters have offered detailed and clear exposés of the nature and various treatment modalities of obsessive-compulsive disorder (OCD). However, several questions relating to the internal cohesiveness of the syndrome, OCD's relationship to depressive disorder and other anxiety disorders, and the significance of advances in current therapeutics remain. These are fascinating and problematic areas requiring further elucidation, and an attempt will be made here to discuss them as well as to suggest possibilities for future research.

MATIG MAVISSAKALIAN, SAMUEL TURNER, and LARRY MICHELSON • Western Psychiatric Institute and Clinic, University of Pittsburgh School of Medicine, 3811 O'Hara Street, Pittsburgh, Pennsylvania 15213.

In discussing the internal cohesiveness of OCD, several issues require consideration. These include the multiplicity of phenomenological variance of obsessive-compulsive symptoms, the diversity of the functional relationship between obsessive and compulsive phenomena, the unitary formulations of OCD based on empirical observations and theoretical concepts, and finally, the recent introduction of functional classifications that provide the possibility of new directions in the assessment and treatment of OCD.

PHENOMENOLOGICAL VARIANCE

In recent years, many phenomenological studies have accurately delineated the various types and forms of obsessive-compulsive symptoms (Mavissakalian & Barlow, 1981; see also Chapters 1 and 2). Briefly, Akhtar, Wig, Verma, Pershad, and Verma (1975) found that dirt and contamination were the most frequent ideational content of obsessions, followed in descending order by aggression and violence, religion, and sex. These results are in accord with clinical observations and were recently confirmed by Stern and Cobb (1978). Akhtar *et al.* (1975) also described different forms of obsessions that would transcend content as demonstrated in this example:

> A woman who worries about her child's safety might have an obsessive doubt (has something happened to him?), or an obsessive fear (something might happen to him because of my negligence), or an obsessive image (I see him drowning!), or obsessional thinking (if he plays outside he may catch cold, that might turn into pneumonia, and if that goes undiagnosed, then. . .). (p. 345)

The most commonly encountered obsessional forms in their study were, in descending order, doubts, thinking, fears, impulses, and images.

Stern and Cobb (1978), in contrast, aimed at classifying symptomatology into behavioral forms and identified four major and three minor forms. The major forms consisted of cleaning, avoiding, repeating, and checking rituals. Washing (cleaning) and checking also emerged as the major types of compulsive behaviors in a factor analytic study conducted by Hodgson and Rachman (1977). The three minor forms identified by Stern and Cobb (1978) were (a) slowness (of motor action as if they were carried in slow motion); (b) completeness (with the aim of doing things properly); and (c) meticulousness (a concern that objects be arranged in specific order). Stern and Cobb commented that the minor forms contribute to the same clinical problem, which is that single tasks take up much time in the patient's everyday life. Hodgson and Rachman (1977) also identified two minor types of compulsive behaviors. Slowness was characterized by slow repetitive behavior unrelated to anxiety or persistent ruminations. The second, doubting, was characterized by uncertainty concerning the compulsive behavior as well as daily activities.

Relevant to our discussion here are recent findings suggesting that the different types or forms of OCD connote prognostic and demographic differences. To start with, approximately 25% of OCD patients have obsessions without accompanying motoric compulsions, and several authors have reported that absence of compulsive behavior is a favorable prognostic sign (Akhtar et al., 1975; Ingram, 1961a; Lo, 1967). This is, in itself, puzzling because obsessions have been notoriously difficult to treat with behavioral techniques. Furthermore, two studies (Hackman & McLean, 1975; Stern, 1978) have also suggested that obsessional fears might respond better than other obsessional forms to treatment with prolonged exposure. Even more provocative are the differences reported between the two prototypes of motoric compulsions, namely checkers and washers (see Chapter 1). Perhaps the most revealing of these differences is the disproportionate representation of females (4:1) with cleaning/washing compulsions compared to the roughly equal sex ratio in checking compulsions (Rachman & Hodgson, 1981).

Despite these reported differences, the significance of a classification of obsessive-compulsive disorder by specific types is not yet clear, especially because multiple types and forms of obsessions and compulsions are present in a substantial proportion of patients (Akhtar et al., 1975; Hodgson & Rachman, 1977; Stern & Cobb, 1978). However, these studies, in addition to the functional diversity of obsessive-compulsive phenomena to be discussed later, have begun to challenge the unitary conceptualization of OCD.

FUNCTIONAL DIVERSITY

Even when the difficulties posed by the various phenomenological types can be circumvented by focusing on the functional relationship of obsessions and compulsions, one is faced with controversy. That obsessions, whether spontaneous or provoked, are associated with anxiety has been amply demonstrated in carefully conducted behavioral and psychophysiological studies (Boulougouris & Bassiakos, 1973; Boulougouris, Rabavilas, & Stefanis, 1977; Hodgson & Rachman, 1972; Rabavilas & Boulougouris, 1974; Roper & Rachman, 1976; Roper, Rachman & Hodgson, 1973; Stern, Lipsedge, & Marks 1973). The problem is posed by the observation that compulsions, which, in the most part, reduce anxiety/distress and neutralize obsessions, can and do elevate anxiety associated with obsessions (Reed, 1968; Roper et al., 1973; Wolpe, 1958).

Beech and Liddell (1974) have maintained that rituals increase the anxiety/discomfort that accompanies obsessions. An excellent example of an attempt to systematically investigate mood changes accompanying ritualistic behavior was reported by Walker and Beech (1969). Their findings, based on detailed interviewing and direct observation and ratings of mood (hostility, depression, and anxiety), contradicted traditionally held views that compulsions uniformly have an anxiety-reducing function and that one should not interrupt the ritual for fear that this might acutely exacerbate the patient's anxious and dysphoric mood. According to Beech,

> First, there is a strong tendency for the mood of patients to show increasing deterioration as the ritual proceeds, and on a good proportion of occasions the patient will terminate his ritual in a considerably more distressed state than that in which he began. Secondly, as a matter of empirical fact, the interruption of a ritual has a generally beneficial effect upon mood state. (Beech, 1971, pp. 420–421)

Rachman and his associates (see Chapter 1), on the other hand, have conclusively demonstrated that in the majority of washers and checkers the performance of rituals is followed by a decline of the urges to engage in the ritual and a decrease in anxiety/discomfort. However, they also found evidence that on occasion patients experienced increased anxiety/discomfort during the rituals (Roper et al., 1973). Thus, any unitary formulation of OCD should be able to account for this functional diversity and accommodate the fact that compulsions and rituals can produce an increment in anxiety/discomfort.

To complicate matters, rituals can also become autonomous of underlying obsessions or anxiety/distress. Marks, Crowe, Drewe, Young, and Dewhurst (1969) gave an illustration of desynchrony between obsessions and compulsions in that washing rituals were maintained despite the successful desensitization of the contamination fears in their patient. Earlier, Walton and Mather (1963) had hypothesized that disassociations between obsessions and compulsions would be more likely to occur in the chronic stages of the illness. More recently, Rachman (1974) has described 10 patients with "primary obsessional slowness" in whom rituals consisted of spending long periods of time on the simplest of tasks such as showering, brushing teeth, shaving, getting dressed and the like. Of interest is that these extensive rituals seem to have no apparant link to underlying obsessions or to anxiety/discomfort.

UNIFYING CLINICAL CONCEPTS

In the face of such phenomenological and functional diversity, clinicians traditionally have recognized and used certain essential features to diagnose OCD. These have been lucidly defined by Lewis (1966) and are included in the latest diagnostic criteria of the disorder (American Psychiatric Association, 1980). In Lewis's words:

> In this condition, the characteristic feature is that, along with some mental happening, there is an experience of subjective compulsion and of resistance to it. Commonly the mental happening (which may be a fear, an impulse or a preoccupation) is recognized on quiet reflection, as senseless; nevertheless it persists. (p. 1199)

Recent studies, however, have suggested that these traditionally perceived axial syndromal features are not essential features of OCD and that they too may vary among its phenomenological subtypes. For example, Stern and Cobb

(1978) found that only 30% of OCD patients demonstrated great resistance to performing the ritual and that as many as 35% of patients did not recognize the senselessness of their rituals. Similarly, the percentage of patients who always tried to resist was low (14%) in the sample reported by Rachman and Hodgson (1981). Even more revealing was their finding that senselessness and resistance were more commonly associated with checking compulsions than with cleaning compulsions.

Akhtar *et al.* (1975) operationally defined two categories of compulsions and found that 61% of their OCD patients had yielding compulsions (when the compulsive act gave expression to the underlying obsessive urge), but only 6% had controlling compulsions (when the compulsive act tended to divert the underlying obsession). More interestingly, they reported that controlling compulsions were associated with better outcome. Although it is plausible to assume that yielding compulsions connote lack of resistance, it should be stressed that the definitional criteria differ between the studies reported. Rachman and Hodgson (1981) described resistance to the act itself, whereas yielding compulsions were defined in relation to underlying obsession. Furthermore, Rachman and Hodgson cautioned against the difficulties involved in assessing such complex psychological phenomena as resistance and senselessness. Nevertheless, these findings suggest that resistance and senselessness, far from being universal features of OCD, might, in addition, be dependent of phenomenology and related to outcome.

Another major unifying concept in OCD has been provided by the traditional psychoanalytical view, according to which the various types of symptoms are only expressions of the basic "anal-erotic character" manifested by obstinacy, parsimony, and orderliness (Fenichel, 1946; Freud, 1908/1924). In an interesting and informative exercise, Ingram (1961b) compared descriptions of the anal-erotic character with descriptions of obsessive-compulsive personality from authoritative sources and came to the conclusion that they had much in common:

> Although the names selected for the main categories vary slightly, there is agreement on the importance of orderliness, persistence, and rigidity.... The description of the obsessional personality shows a greater emphasis on inconclusiveness and on related fears, doubts and checking activities. This suggests an overlap or continuum between these traits and the symptoms of obsessional illness. (p. 1040)

The studies investigating the relationship of obsessive-compulsive personality and OCD have provided only partial confirmation of this viewpoint. These have been summarized by Black (1974) who revealed that one-fourth to one-third of OCD patients have no evidence of predisposing personality traits. Similarly, a recent comprehensive review of the literature led Pollak (1979) to conclude that "obsessive compulsive personality can be statistically differentiated from obsessive compulsive symptomatology through factor analysis" (p. 238).

In the search for essential obsessional traits, indecisiveness has received an all-important place, not only in obsessive-compulsive personality but also in OCD (Makhlouf-Norris & Norris, 1972; Reed, 1968). Indecisiveness (and dysphoria) has also been a critical element in Beech's view of obsessive-compulsive disorder and a prime explanatory hinge for anxiety-augmenting compulsions (Beech, 1971; Beech & Liddell, 1974). Thus, it would seem, when the patient cannot decide when to stop his or her ritual and continues to perform it over and over, that this would cause deterioration of mood and increase anxiety discomfort. As was discussed before, this may explain some, but clearly not all, situations. Furthermore, it appears that indecisiveness and doubting are more prominent in checking compulsions than in cleaning compulsions (Rachman & Hodgson, 1981).

Before closing the discussion on personality, it may well be worth returning to the minor behavioral forms of completeness and meticulousness discussed by Stern and Cobb (1978) that seem to create a common clinical picture called *primary obsessional slowness* (Rachman, 1974). These patients, it should be reminded, perform prolonged rituals unprovoked by obsessions and without any clear relationship to anxiety discomfort. It is therefore tempting to assume that this phenomenological variant of obsessive-compulsive symptoms might represent hypertrophic obsessive-compulsive personality traits. However, even if the continuum between obsessive-compulsive personality and primary obsessional slowness is unequivocally established, it would be difficult to generalize from this minor and infrequently encountered phenomenological variant to OCD in general. Lewis's (1936) early observations in this regard still hold true and lucidly summarize the relationship of obsessive-compulsive personality and symptoms:

> Of course, may obsessionals have shown excessive cleanliness, orderliness, pedantry, conscientiousness, uncertainty, inconclusive ways of thinking and acting. These are sometimes obsessional symptoms themslves, sometimes character traits devoid of any immediate experience of subjective compulsion. They are, however, especially in the later case, just as commonly found among patients who never have an obsessional neurosis, but who get an agitated melancholia.... I have verified this on a large number of patients at the Maudsley Hospital. The traits are also, of course, common among healthy people. They are conversely, sometimes undiscoverable in the previous personality of patients who now have a severe obsessional neurosis. (p. 328)

RECENT FUNCTIONAL FORMULATIONS

The phenomenological classification of OCD has yielded few but important differences, the full clinical and nosological implications of which await further investigations. On the other hand, the search for a unifying concept encompassing all phenomenological forms has not been entirely successful. The major shortcoming of these descriptive classificatory schemes is that they are, by definition, structurally static and hence do not do justice to the fluidity and dynamic interplay of obsessive-compulsive phenomena. Nor do they account for their fluctuations of severity or changes in pattern encountered in the natural course or during treatment. In order to develop a viable unitary conceptualization of OCD, the classificatory formulation needs to go beyond the mere subdivision of obsessive-compulsive phenomena into different forms and content as well as to account for their functional diversity.

A first attempt at such a classification was offered by Lewis (1957):

> Obsessions can be conveniently divided into primary and secondary. An example would be first, the insistent feeling that she is dirty—that is the primary phenomenon. And then there is the impulse to wash—the secondary phenomenon developed in order to obtain relief from the primary disturbance. The second phenomenon can be regarded as defensive, and aimed at preventing or relieving tension. They can themselves be obsessional, that is, the patient has to struggle against them and may indeed develop defensive rituals or tricks against them in turn; or they may remain neutral and unresisted, they may indeed be prized for their protective efficacy. (p. 158)

A clear implication in Lewis's definition is the dynamic concept that compulsions that begin with a defensive purpose can become the source of anxiety requiring ''defensive rituals and tricks against them." In other words, a secondary phenomenon (compulsion) can itself become a second primary phenomenon (obsession). As will be seen, this insight might well bridge the controversy between anxiety-inducing and anxiety-reducing compulsions.

Equally essential to a unitary functional formulation of OCD is the notion of functional equivalence between overt and covert obsessive-compulsive phenomena. Rachman (1976) has thus made a distinction between the thoughts that act as "noxious stimuli" (obsessions) and thoughts that attempt to neutralize them. Furthermore, he has proposed that we assume a functional equivalence between compulsive checking and cleaning and the compulsive thoughts on the basis that all of these constitute attempts to neutralize obsessions. More recent formulations (Foa & Tillmanns 1980; Mavissakalian, 1979) have further proposed that obsessive-compulsive phenomena be classified according to their psychophysiological effect rather than their intended function. Thus, obsessions have been defined as phenomena that induce anxiety, whereas compulsions are phenomena that reduce anxiety discomfort and neutralize obsessions. As was reviewed earlier (cf. Chapters 1 and 2), there is ample empirical support for such a definition.

In addition to its parsimony, the functional formulation has the advantage of providing a rational and uniform basis for the analysis and treatment of obsessive-compulsive phenomena along the lines described by Foa and associates (Chapter 2). Thus, according to this formulation, anxiety-augmenting compulsions would be considered functional obsessions and appropriately targeted by the technique of prolonged exposure, whereas compulsions that are anxiety-reducing would be treated by response prevention. In the case of the functionally autonomous rituals, however, one would not think of prolonged exposure nor of response prevention as the treatment modalities of choice. Rather, a completely different approach, perhaps consisting of shaping, pacing, and prompting, in short, of symptom scheduling, might be more appropriate (Mavissakalian, 1979; Rachman, 1974). The new directions for the behavioral treatments that this functional classification generates will be discussed in greater detail later. An additional advantage of the functional classification is the possibility of utilizing changes in the dynamic interaction between obsessions and compulsions in the assessment of different stages of severity and chronicity of this disorder (Mavissakalian, 1979).

According to this formulation, obsessions are the starting point, that is, the primary phenomena, that set the obsessive-compulsive disorder in motion. Rachman and de Silva (1978) have reported that obsessions, defined as repetitive, intrusive, unwanted thoughts, are common occurrences in "normals" (cf. Chapter 1). However, obsessions of OCD patients are differentiated from normal obsessions in that the former last longer, produce more discomfort, and are more ego alien, more strongly resisted, harder to dismiss, and provoke more urges to neutralize. Whatever the reasons for the tenacity of obsessions, the OCD patient thus afflicted engages in compulsive behavior to neutralize the obsessions and to find relief from the associated anxiety discomfort.

This state of affairs (obsessions plus anxiety-reducing compulsions) seems to represent a relatively stable stage of the disorder that may well explain the long durations typically encountered before the patient seeks treatment. It has been our clinical impression that most patients seek help when previously successful compulsions fail, that is, when OCD enters a new and unstable stage. The patients often state that what used to work does not any longer. They find themselves to be more anxious, and they report experiencing more frequent and intense obsessions that they are unable to neutralize as before and that their compulsive behavior has become itself a source of discomfort. We would like to suggest that Beech's conceptualization of obsessive-compulsive disorder, greatly emphasizing the indecisiveness, doubting, and increasing dysphoria, would eminently describe this stage of the disorder. It remains a challenge for future research to determine whether dysphoric mood brings upon increasing indecisiveness that obsessionalizes the previously successful compulsive behavior, or whether it is the failure of compulsive behavior to neutralize the obsessions successfully and the subsequent frustrating struggle that leads to the dysphoria. What is certain is that both are intimately associated upon the presentation of the patients. Indeed, Foa (1979) and Foa *et al.* (Chapter 2) have recently found evidence for the impedence of habituation to take place in depressed OCD patients. Furthermore, the literature suggests such an intimate relationship between depression and obsessive-compulsive disorder that it will be discussed in greater detail under a separate heading.

The recent phenomenological and functional classifications of obsessive-compulsive phenomena should be taken as hypothetical suggestions awaiting empirical testing. They attest to the continuing puzzle presented by the nature of obsessive-compulsive disorder and represent ways of rationally ordering the richness of the phenomena. Eventually, a classification system based on the unitary concepts inherent in the functional formulations and incorporating changes in mood and psychophysiological arousal might evolve to accurately reflect the dynamic nature of obsessive-compulsive disorder. Because of the importance of these dynamic factors, we will turn now to the discussion of the relationship between OCD and the other anxiety disorders on the one hand and depressive dis-

order on the other. With the exception of functionally autonomous rituals that possess so many unusual features that their
inclusion in the body of OCD should be seriously questioned,
a somewhat arbitrary yet necessary unitary view of obsessive-
compulsive phenomena will be adopted for this purpose.

RELATION TO ANXIETY DISORDERS

The question of whether OCD is associated with other
psychiatric disorders has served as an impetus for much con-
jecture, hypothesizing, and debate. Conceptual and theoretical models of etiology, phenomenology, and treatment have
historically clashed when examining this question. Unfortunately, the paucity of large-scale epidemiological studies of
the major anxiety disorders, diagnosed according to uniform
specific and objective criteria, prevents accurate assessment of
the prevalence and incidence of these disorders, including
obsessive-compulsive disorder (Sartorius, 1980). Furthermore,
the hidden nature of obsessional states, the reluctance of
many patients to seek treatment, and probably the stability of
the disorder, as discussed before, account for the reported rarity of OCD in clinical practice.

The evidence from family and genetic studies, although
pointing toward the familial incidence of obsessive-compulsive
disorder, has revealed a substantial overlap among the different anxiety disorders in the history and families of patients
(Rachman & Hodgson 1981). In lieu of a specific genetic in-
heritance for OCD, the literature suggests that a genetic
predisposition to neurotic illness, also called anxiety prone-
ness, may underlie the major anxiety disorders (Carey & Gottesman, 1981; Shields, 1978). Furthermore, psychophysiological studies reveal that anxiety neurotics, agoraphobics, and

obsessive-compulsive patients are characterized by increased levels of arousal that distinguish them from "normals" (Kelly, 1980; Lader, 1978). This would suggest that anxiety disorders may represent different levels of complexity and severity of the same basic process.

A certain degree of blurring between panic disorder and agoraphobia is readily apparent in the *Diagnostic and Statistical Manual of Mental Disorders* (DSM-III). Also apparent is the fact that panic attacks consist of sudden discrete episodes of exacerbations in the somatic and psychic components of generalized anxiety disorder. These typically include intense apprehension, feelings of unreality, terror, and the fear of dying or going crazy or doing something out of control. They are often accompanied by an autonomic storm marked by palpitations, chest pain, dyspnea, choking and smothering sensations, paresthesia, sweating, trembling or shaking, and dizziness or faintness. Panic attacks apparently come from nowhere, although most often during stressful situations (grief is common) or with general anxiety disorder in the background. Such panic attacks are frequent in, and invariably mark the onset of, agoraphobia and lead to precautionary measures to avoid experiencing repeated attacks. Although a cardinal symtom of agoraphobia is avoidance of multiple situations, on closer examination, the patient's central fear seems to be the fear of panicking in these situations. This contrasts with simple phobias that represent a specific response to circumscribed situations where the fear relates to the situation's impact on the person. That is, the source of danger is external and inherent in the situation rather than, as in the case of agoraphobia, a fear of one's own reactions in these situations. Furthermore, in simple phobias, there are no signs of generalized chronic anxiety or spontaneous panic attacks or depersonalization phenomena as in the case of agoraphobia.

The fear of panicking in agoraphobics is also similar to the fear of losing control of obsessive-compulsive patients. Thus, in both conditions, external stimuli, whether a knife or a crowded place, precipitate a more central internal fear of losing control with the negative consequences of physical, mental, or social annihilation. Obsessional thoughts, as is well known, occur spontaneously, as do panic attacks. In both instances, the patient struggles to suppress the intruder or to take precautionary or restorative measures. Indeed, phobic avoidance is as common in obsessive-compulsive disorder as in agoraphobia. Furthermore, compulsive behaviors share a functional equivalence in that they aim at neutralizing, that is, preventing or undoing the obsessionally feared consequences, and thus they can be conceptualized as active avoidance. Such functionally equivalent behavior is often seen in agoraphobics as witnessed by their frequent calls for reassurance and their checking on the whereabouts of trusted people for security cues. Likewise, their compulsive carrying of tranquilizers, even though they know it is silly, that they will not take one and that it rarely helps anyway, their rigidly mapped itinerary dotted with security cues from which they dare not deviate, the specified places where they sit in churches or restaurants, the specific times they visit stores, all point to this phenomenon.

In brief, the major difference between anxiety neurosis (or panic disorder), agoraphobia and obsessive-compulsive disorder seems to be that in the last two conditions the patient attempts to reduce, and temporarily succeeds in so doing, the anxiety attacks and the feared consequence of losing control, whether this is in the form of fainting, embarrassing oneself, being irrevocably contaminated, hurting others, or in some way being hurt oneself. In agoraphobia, the instigator is panic or depersonalization, whereas in obsessive-compulsive disorder it consists of obsessions, as discussed earlier. Learning theory further postulates that the reduction of anxiety acts as a negative reinforcer and thus strengthens and maintains the avoidance or compulsive behavior. Habitual avoidance, on the other hand, precludes any chance of extinction of phobic anxiety or obsessions.

It is interesting that the effectiveness of behavioral treatments has hinged on essentially reversing these patterns. Exposure to stimuli provoking anxiety by preventing escape behavior, leads to extinction of phobic anxiety or obsessions. It is no less interesting that the so-called spontaneous panic attacks of agoraphobics also respond to exposure treatments thus underscoring similarities between panic and phobic anxiety in agoraphobics. However, most agoraphobics or obsessive-compulsive patients are left with a chronic level of generalized anxiety and an avoidant attitude reiminiscent of generalized anxiety disorder. Thus, one can tentatively suggest that panic disorder, agoraphobia, and obsessive-compulsive disorder may represent phenomenological variants of anxiety disorders that share a common and probably genetically determined psychophysiological substrate.

Confirmation of these speculations through rigorously conducted epidemiologic, family, and genetic studies of these disorders is needed to justify their common classification under anxiety disorders. Furthermore, given the fact that learning theory provides an adequate model for the maintenance of symptoms and behavior therapy successfully removes them, it would be misleading to build models of anxiety disorders based solely on genetic or biological mechanisms. Thus, Seligman's (1971) preparedness theory offers an intriguing bridge by stating that certain phobias, for example dirt or contamination, are more commonly reported than other fears due to the selectivity or preparedness of certain stimuli to be more

easily conditioned in contrast to what would be expected on
the basis of random conditioning to the patient's environment,
for example, the "equipotentiality premise" (Rachman, 1977;
Rachman & Seligman, 1976; Seligman, 1970, 1971). Recognizing the disproportionate incidence of certain types of obsessions, compulsions, and fears, certain associations appear to
be more easily acquired. Other stimuli may only become "conditioned" after repeated continuous associations of the unconditioned stimuli (UCS) with the aversive stimuli. Furthermore,
as noted by Seligman (1970), the prepared phobias may be
more resistant to extinction and may operate via noncognitive
channels such as biologic or genetic mechanisms. Seligman
and Hager (1972) also note that those situations are objects
that impact upon the potential survival of the organism and
are the ones most likely to show preparedness and to become
phobically conditioned.

Although there are many unresolved conceptual issues
regarding preparedness theory, one of the more promising ex-
trapolations involves the hypothesized resistance prepared
phobias would have to treatment. However, de Silva, Rachman, and Seligman (1977), in a retrospective study of phobic
and OCD patients, found that the preparedness quality of the
patient's symptoms had little impact upon their resistance or
extinction in clinical outcome. However, as noted by the
authors, the homogeneous and somewhat restricted sample
of severe patients may have obscured differences between the
unprepared and prepared phobics. Nevertheless, de Silva *et
al.* concluded that the preparedness concept may not be useful in predicting the outcome of either OCD or phobic patients.

Recently, there has been an increasing recognition of the
possible role of cognitive factors such as attributions, belief
systems, and expectations in mediating OCD phenomena.

Clinical states including perfectionism, overestimation of harm, dichotomous thinking, deficient cognitive problem-solving strategies, and catastrophic ideation are readily apparent to those who have worked extensively with OCD patients. Unfortunately, few studies have moved beyond this anecdotal level of observation and empirically examined the specific role of these cognitive, mediational, and/or problem-solving strategies among OCD patients. Future efforts in this area may prove fruitful in two specific subareas. First, a thorough assessment of OCD patients should incorporate some index of the patient's cognitive coping style, attributions, expectation of harm, and catastrophizations. This would provide both treatment-planning data as well as serve as a baseline against which clinicians could ascertain the efficacy of their intervention. Second, the mapping of cognitive schemas and information-processing strategies might provide invaluable data leading to more effective intervention in the future. As noted by Foa *et al.* in Chapter 2, the need for a predictive model cannot be overstated.

The absence of cognitive and psychophysiological assessments of OCD patients is readily apparent when reviewing the literature. Unfortunately, theoretical, conceptual, and clinical models of etiology and treatment cannot be fully addressed, given this omission. Future efforts are needed to assess OCD, using a more comprehensive monitoring strategy that enables a finer grained analysis of behavioral, physiological, and cognitive dimensions of functioning. This will allow for important phenomena such as synchrony/desynchrony, concordance/disconcordance, and habituation to be studied more systematically. Research delineating these parameters of therapeutic efficacy are gradually emerging as investigators specifically examine the relationship between mood, cognitive, motoric, and physiological response domains. Moreover, the controlled manipulation of behavioral (e.g., exposure vs. response prevention) and pharmacologic treatments offers much promise toward the elucidation of response selectivity as well as the relationship between mood, behavioral, cognitive, and physiological dimensions of the disorder. Before discussing the implications for therapy, however, let us briefly turn to the relationship of OCD to depression.

RELATION TO DEPRESSION

In several places in this volume, the close relationship between depression and OCD has been mentioned and discussed already (see Chapters 1, 2, and 5). The reader is also referred to the excellent critical review presented by Rachman and Hodgson (1980) of this puzzling relationship. Clearly, well-controlled clinical and family studies of rigorously diagnosed primary depressive and primary OCD patients will do much toward clarifying important aspects of this relationship.

Recently, a potentially fruitful avenue in studying the relationship of depression and OCD has been reported by Insel and associates. These investigators found that 9 out of 14 OCD patients studied with all-night sleep EEG (Insel, Gillin, Moore, Mendelson, Loewenstein, & Murphy, 1982) and 6 out of 16 OCD patients tested with the Dexamethasone Suppression Test (Insel, Kalin, Guttmacher, Cohen, & Murphy, 1982), had an abnormal response typical of depressive disorder. Although a number of methodological confounds prohibit definitive conclusions from being drawn, that is, most patients met criteria of major depression, these findings suggest the possibility of a common psychobiological link between OCD and depression and warrant systematic replication efforts.

A common biological substrate between the two disorders

is also suggested by the recent successes in the treatment of OCD with antidepressant drugs. It comes as no surprise, therefore, that investigators have been interested in the question of whether antidepressants have specific antiobsessional effects above and beyond their antidepressant action (see Chapter 5). Unfortunately, the issue is highly controversial, and two of the better controlled studies have reported contradictory findings. Thoren, Asberg, Cronholm, Jornestedt, & Traskman (1980) found that neither diagnosis nor degree of depression was associated with response to clomipramine, whereas Marks, Stenn, Mawson, Cobb, & McDonald (1980) found that antiobsessional effect was noted mainly in patients with high pretreatment depression scores. Recent findings in our center did not lend support to the claim that tricyclics possess a specific antiobsessional effect. In this study (Mavissakalian & Michelson, 1983), not only change in obsessive-compulsive symptoms paralleled change in depression and anxiety, suggesting a global beneficial effect of the drugs and a synchronous pattern of change between these various symptomatologies, but it appeared that responders had substantially higher initial Hamilton Depression ratings compared to nonresponders. Because numbers are very small, these results need cautious interpretation. Furthermore, the general patholytic effect of antidepressant drugs as well as the high degrees of correlations between the various symptom ratings point to the limitations of studies trying to elucidate the mechanism of action of antidepressants on symptomatic grounds alone. On the other hand, there have been promising suggestive indications of a biochemical differentiation between the antiobsessional and antidepressant actions of clomipramine.

Thoren, Asberg, Bertilsson, Mellstrom, Sjoqvista, and Traskman (1980) reported that improvement in obsessive-compulsive symptoms was associated with the reduction of

CSF-5-hydroxindoleacetic acid but not to levels of hydroxy-3-methoxphenol glycol (the respective metabolites of serotonin and noradrenaline). In addition, Stern, Marks, Mawson, and Luscombe (1980) reported that plasma clomipramine concentration (a powerful inhibitor of serotonin reuptake) was related to improvement in rituals, whereas the plasma N-desmethylclomipramine level (the active metabolite of clomipramine that primarily inhibits noradrenaline reuptake) was related to outcome of depression. These studies therefore suggest a prominent role for serotonin in mediating improvement of obsessive-compulsive symptoms and suggest a biochemical differentiation between the antiobsessional and antidepressive effects of clomipramine in this disorder (see also Chapter 5). Of considerable research interest are the recently developed antidepressants that selectively act on the serotonergic and noradrenergic systems and thus provide an excellent opportunity to dissect pharmacologically the various effects of antidepressants and their possible differential mediation across neurotransmitter systems.

A recent pilot study with fluoxetine hydrochloride, a selective serotonergic agent, was reported by Turner, Jacob, Beidel, and Himmelhoch (1984). Ten obsessive-compulsive patients meeting DSM-III criteria were treated over a 3-month period. Patients were begun on 20 mg of fluoxetine and gradually increased to a maximum of 80 mg. A battery of self-report and clinical rating scales were employed to assess pre- and posttreatment functioning. There was a slow improvement over the treatment period in self-reported distress and frequency of obsessions, frequency of rituals, amount of time spent ritualizing, and amount of time being preoccupied with obsessive thoughts. The change in time spent ritualizing, time spent obsessing, and self-reported distress level all reached statistical significance from pre- to posttreatment. Similarly, significant changes were obtained on a number of self-report inventories. These data are particularly impressive because they suggest fluoxetine had some direct effect on the obsessions and compulsions *per se*. Although this sample was too small to allow for examination of subtypes, the authors concluded that those patients evidencing the severest level of depression appeared to respond the most to the drug.

Undoubtedly, more research along clinical, psychobiological, and pharmacological dimensions will focus on the relationship between depression and OCD, and, indeed, all other anxiety disorders. In addition, long-term prospective followup studies of obsessive-compulsive patients will be invaluable in studying the clinical observations that OCD and depression commonly overlap, yet often run independent and desynchronous courses.

TREATMENT

In this section, we will limit our discussion primarily to behavioral and drug treatments and highlight areas of controversy, inconsistencies, possible outcome predictors, and avenues for future research. The question of how obsessive-compulsives fare in treatment has never been satisfactorily answered. The prevailing clinical lore even today is that obsessionals do not respond as well in treatment with respect to short- or long-term outcome, regardless of the intervention employed. Thus, obsessive-compulsives are sometimes passed from therapist to therapist, and sometimes, as in the case of a recent referral to our clinic, are told their disorder is untreatable.

In one of the earliest reports, Lewis (1936) noted that among 50 obsessionals treated with various modalities, 32%

were described as quite normal, 14% were much improved, 10% relapsed, and 34% were unchanged over a 5-year period. Nineteen years later, Kringlen (1965) reported a 13- to 20-year follow-up of a sample of patients comprised of obsessionals and phobics with additional unspecified symptoms. Of the surviving patients at follow-up, roughly 75% were unchanged, whereas about 25% were judged to be much improved.

In the same year, Grimshaw (1965) reported the follow-up of 100 patients over a period of 1 to 14 years. A variety of treatments (psychotherapy, supportive therapy, ECT, leucotomy) was employed. Grimshaw concluded that there was a good response to about 64% of the cases with respect to symptoms. Accepting the improvement rates of 25%, 64%, and 46% (combining 32% and 14% from Lewis, 1936), the outcome does not appear to be quite as poor as predicted, but these figures do indicate the resistance of this condition to treatment.

Sifneos (Chapter 3) reported that a short-term psychoanalytic procedure was effective in treating obsessive-compulsives. However, it is questionable as to whether the group of patients treated by Sifneos would meet current accepted criteria (DSM-III) for obsessive-compulsive disorder. From the description provided, it appears that these patients might be more accurately described as compulsive personality disorder, according to DSM-III criteria. The relationship of compulsive personality characteristics to the actual disorder was discussed earlier, and, as noted, the relationship is not a consistent one. Thus, it is difficult to evaluate the utility of the treatment described by Sifneos in treating obsessive-compulsive disorder (see Chapter 3).

In reviews of behavioral interventions (Chapter 2), treatment effectiveness was reported to be in the 70% range. This represents a significant advance in the management of this condition. This figure is gleaned from a rather large literature, and the criteria for improvement are not always clearly specified or calculated in the same fashion. However, the studies on which these figures are based tend to have employed subjects with overt ritualistic behavior (mostly washing/cleaning, checking, and combinations of both), giving confidence to diagnostic integrity. Moreover, many of the reports contain objective data to support their claims of improvement. In most studies, some variant of exposure treatment and response prevention comprised the treatment strategy. Thus, in these reports, an encouraging picture with respect to treatment is portrayed. Moreover, specific therapeutic strategies are noted to account for the results.

Mawson, Marks, and Ramm (1982) followed 37 patients over a 2-year period who had been treated with clomipramine and/or varying amounts of exposure treatment. These authors reported that their patients were significantly improved over pretreatment at the 2-year assessment on every measure. This report is noteworthy in that a good pre-post assessment battery consisting of self-report and rating scales was included. With respect to prediction of treatment, the central finding was that the more prolonged the exposure, the better the outcome. There was no relation to outcome for such widely studied variables as level of depression or anxiety. This report provided strong support for the long-term efficacy of exposure treatment.

In another report, Kirk (1983) described the results of a sample of 36 patients followed up over a period of 1 to 5 years. The study is somewhat problematic in that about half of the patients were treated with drugs and 4 received some inpatient treatment in addition to outpatient therapy. Also, some patients received home-based exposure, and some were aided in their treatment regimen by relatives, whereas others were not. The treatment consisted primarily of response prevention and flooding, and, to a lesser extent, thought stopping and relaxation. There was also some assertive training, marital counseling, and problem solving. Hence, the treatment might best be described as a comprehensive behavioral approach. Judgment of outcome was based on global ratings with the following results: 81% of the patients were judged to have made good progress; 81% did not require additional referral during the 1 to 5 year period; and only 15 cases had required additional behavioral treatment. Although this report does not provide support for specific types of intervention, it is most encouraging when viewed in the context of prognosis for obsessive-compulsive patients.

Taken together, the previously mentioned studies suggest that the outlook is not dismal for obsessional patients. To the contrary, the improvement ratings obtained with exposure and response prevention are comparable to the treatment of other anxiety states (e.g., agoraphobia) by behavioral strategies. Moreover, it appears that these improvements are not temporary but last at least 1 to 5 years without significant rates of recurrence. Yet, numerous other procedures such as pacing and shaping strategies, relaxation therapy, and marital or family intervention have also been used singularly and in conjunction with exposure and response prevention. In our clinical experience, additional treatment is frequently necessary. Thus, it is unclear how much the use of these additional strategies contributes to long-term outcome. Stressful life experiences are seen as important in influencing the course of OCD. In fact, a diathesis—stress model has been suggested as an etiological model (e.g., Carey & Gottesman, 1981; Turner & Beidel, 1984). It would seem that when attempts are made to help the patient cope with life stresses and prepare her or him to cope with future stressful events, better long-term maintenance can be expected. It is to be hoped that greater attention will be devoted to this issue in the future.

Pharmacological treatments have also shown promise in the obsessional states, and these treatments were reviewed in Chapter 5. The drugs most often studied are antidepressant agents, and there is continuing controversy as to whether they achieve their effects through mood elevation or whether they have specific antiobsessive-compulsive properties as previously noted (Mavissakalian, 1983).

There is considerable evidence that clomipramine, a potent inhibitor of serotonin reuptake, has significant beneficial effects in treating obsessions. Although it is unclear what the mechanism of action of clomipramine is, and a report by Insel, Gillin, Moore, Mendelson, Loewenstein, and Murphy *et al.* (1982) casts some doubt on a central role for serotonin, there is support for the utility of this drug in obsessional states. However, the available literature suggests that relapse occurs fairly rapidly following discontinuation of the drug. Also, side effects can be problematic with clomipramine (Rachman, Cobb, Grey, MacDonald, Mawson, Sartory, & Stern, 1979), although it is still unclear if side effects and/or relapse are associated with specific patient characteristics. Clarification of these issues await further study.

COMBINED TREATMENTS

Although there are a number of single-case and small-group studies demonstrating the effectiveness of combined drug and behavioral treatments (Turner, Hersen, Bellack, Androsik & Capparell, 1979; Turner, Hersen, Bellack, Andrasik, & Capparell, 1980), to date the best controlled group study (Rachman *et al.*, 1979) found no additive effect for combined treatment. However, Foa *et al.* (Chapter 2) have suggested that severely depressed patients do not habituate within flooding sessions and may well not respond to exposure treatment until their affective state is relieved. Interestingly, in a recently completed study (Turner *et al.*, 1984), dramatic additional response to a 10-day regimen of exposure *in vivo* and response prevention following 3 months of treatment with fluoxetine hydrochloride was obtained. Indeed, the results indicated that priming patients with the drug may have potentiated the effects of exposure to the point that continuing booster sessions were not required at follow-up. Therefore, we believe the use of combined pharmacological and behavioral intervention is worthy of further research, particularly in regard to the thoroughness of recovery. Whether such a procedure is related to long-term outcome, however, remains to be seen.

PREDICTOR VARIABLES

The examination of predictor variables in obsessive-compulsive disorder has not been conducted in a rigorous fashion (Chapter 1). Primarily, the work that has been done is related to anxiety and depression. Foa *et al.* (Chapter 2) presented data to suggest that high levels of depression are predictive of poor response to behavioral interventions. In fact, treatment with antidepressants prior to exposure treatment is recommended for individuals with high levels of depression (Chapter 5). Our own clinical experience is supportive of this position. However, explicit data have not been put forth, nor are there data to support the premise that this procedure will affect long-term outcome.

The interest in depression does not stop here, however. Depression provides a significant problem in the diagnosis of obsessive disorder. According to DSM-III, if criteria for major depression are met, then that diagnosis must be made. Yet, in many instances depression appears to be a secondary feature occurring long after the appearance of the obsessional disorder. Improvement in depression has been reported following behavioral treatment (e.g., Turner *et al.*, 1979, 1980), and we have observed this to occur on a clinical basis. Yet, it would be interesting to know what level of depression remains when obsessions and compulsions are eliminated, what its course is if present, whether, the initial depression level is related to its continued presence, and whether or not it is predictive of long-term outcome.

Aside from the decrease in anxiety associated with performance of compulsive acts, it is unclear just what role anxiety plays in obsessional states. In a study designed to examine physiological arousal, Rabavilas, Boulougouris, Perissaki, and Stefanis (1979) administered propranolol to OCD patients. Although there were reductions in physiological arousal as expected, clinical ratings of symptomatology did not decrease, and patients did not report themselves as less anxious or more content when using the drug. Ananth (Chapter 5) also suggests that, although certain pharmacological preparations may reduce arousal levels, they do not necessarily decrease the primary symptoms of obsessions and compulsions. Does this imply that arousal does not have a primary role in the disorder? Although we do not know the answer to this question, the preceding findings are consistent with other reports in the literature. For example, Lader (1974) demonstrated that, although arousal and anxiety are often confused, level of physiological arousal does not always correlate with the subjectively perceived experience of anxiety. In a clinical demonstration, anxiety patients treated with diazepam evidenced a decreased level of physiological arousal but no concomitant changes in perceived level of anxiety (Lader, 1974). Exactly what bearing this has on the relationship of anxiety to obsessional states and as a possible predictor variable for treatment awaits empirical clarification. The work described in Chapter 2, however, suggests the possibility that high anxiety/arousal levels may hinder the process of habituation.

Indeed, Foa *et al.* (Chapter 2) presented data to suggest that habituation to feared stimuli is a necessary, but not sufficient, predictor of response to behavioral treatment between sessions. They reported that in no instance was between-sessions habituation obtained in the absence of within-sessions habituation, although within-sessions habituation did not guarantee between-sessions success. Yet, whether or not a patient habituates within sessions might well predict outcome. At this time, there are no definitive data regarding this variable and subsequent short- and long-term response to treatment.

Other variables worth investigating would be the prognostic implications of phenomenologic and psychobiologic characteristics associated with OCD. Thus, it has been suggested that resistance and senselessness, once considered central variables in the diagnosis of obsessional states, are not always present in OCD patients. Whether or not the level of resistance and degree of perceived senselessness have prognostic value, therefore, is worth investigating. In our clinical experience, patients with both features tend to require less response-prevention supervision, that is, they can often prevent themselves when instructed to do so.

Similarly, although it is clear that not all individuals who develop OCD have compulsive personalities, it is not certain whether or not such premorbid personality traits are related to outcome in OCD. Finally, the application of external validating psychobiological criteria (Akiskal, 1980), such as those currently utilized in the more advanced field of affective disorders, may not only provide important predictive cues as to outcome but may also help further elucidate the nature of the disorder.

ASSESSMENT

The issue of assessment in the treatment of obsessive-compulsive disorder is an important one. The emphasis placed in each of the preceding chapters for the accurate screening and assessment of patients eloquently attests to this fact. Hence, a complete discussion of assessment will not be repeated here (see Mavissakalian & Barlow, 1981). Suffice it to say that assessment is of critical concern to our understanding of the condition as well as to the proper evaluation of treatment outcome.

One of the primary weaknesses of most of the drug studies and some of the behavioral studies is that they fail to assess the effects of treatment on obsessions and compulsions separately. There is a general tendency to employ global rating scales and, in many instances, exclusively self-reported questionnaires possessing questionable psychometric properties. The failure to measure the primary symptoms of OCD in a reliable and valid manner is particularly relevant in drug studies because antidepressants are expected to affect mood, and global ratings of improvement can undoubtedly be a direct reflection of improved mood.

Similarly, it is difficult to assess how much effect improvement in mood, obsessions, and compulsions have on overall social functioning. Little attention has been given to specific assessment in this area. Yet, it is a vital part of the picture in determining the value of any successful treatment. Because stress has been raised as having possible etiological connota-

tions as well as being related to recurrence of symptoms following treatment (Turner & Beidel, 1984), it is somewhat surprising that so little has been done in this area. There is a
considerable literature on the measurement of life events in
depressive disorder (Monroe, 1982a, 1982b) with many possibilities of application in OCD and in investigations of their
relationship.

It is evident that the complexity of obsessive-compulsive
disorder requires a monumental assessment undertaking if
clarity is to be gleaned from current confusions, contradic-
tions, and unexplained findings. The problem is somewhat aggravated by the rarity of the condition, making it difficult for
one center to obtain a sufficient number of subjects to conduct
appropriate designs and analyses. Multicenter studies with
OCD should be given more serious consideration. Moreover,
careful selection of assessment instruments and strategies
designed to explore some of the areas delineated in this chapter, and indeed in the entire volume, will, it is hoped, advance
our understanding of the complexities of obsessive-compulsive
disorder.

References

Akhtar, S., Wig, N. N., Verma, V. J., Pershad, D., & Verma, S. K. A
phenomenological analysis of symptoms in obsessive-compulsive neurosis.
British Journal of Psychiatry, 1975, 127, 342–348.
Akiskal, H. External validating criteria for psychiatric diagnosis: Their appli-
cation in affective disorder. Journal of Clinical Psychiatry, 1980, 41(12), 6–15.
American Psychiatric Association. Diagnostic and statistical manual of mental dis-
orders (3rd ed.). Washington, DC: American Psychiatric Association, 1980.
Beech, H. R. Ritualistic activity in obsessional patients. Journal of Psychosomatic
Research, 1971, 15, 417–422.
Beech, H. R., & Liddell, A. Decision making, mood states, and ritualistic be-
havior among obsessional patients. In H. R. Beech (Ed.) Obsessional states.
London: Methuen, 1974.

Black, A. The natural history of obsessional patients. In H. R. Beech (Ed.), *Obsessional states*. London: Methuen, 1974.

Boulougouris, J. C., & Bassiakos, L. Prolonged flooding in cases with obsessive-compulsive neuroses. *Behaviour Research and Therapy*, 1973, *11*, 227-231.

Boulougouris, J. C., Rabavilas, A. D., & Stefanis, C. Psychophysiological responses in obsessive-compulsive patients. *Behaviour Research and Therapy*, 1977, *15*, 221-230.

Carey, G., & Gottesman, I. I. Twin and family studies of anxiety, phobic and obsessive disorders. In D. F. Klein & J. Rabkin (Eds.), *Anxiety: New research and changing concepts*. New York: Raven, 1981.

de Silva, P., Rachman, S., & Seligman, M. Prepared phobias and obsessions: Therapeutic outcome. *Behaviour Research and Therapy*, 1977, *15*, 54-77.

Fenichel, O. *The psychoanalytic theory of neurosis*. London: Routledge & Kegan Paul, 1946.

Foa, E. B. Failure in treating obsessive-compulsives. *Behaviour Research and Therapy*, 1979, *17*, 169-176.

Foa, E. G., & Tillmanns, A. The treatment of obsessive-compulsive neurosis. In A. Goldstein & E. G. Foa (Eds.), *Handbook of behavioral interventions: A clinical guide*. New York: Wiley, 1980.

Freud, S. Character and anal erotism. *Collected Papers*, (Vol. 2). Hogarth Press, 1924. (Originally published, 1908.)

Grimshaw, L. The outcome of obsessive disorder: A follow-up study of 100 cases. *British Journal of Psychiatry*, 1965, *111*, 1051-1056.

Hackman, A., & McLean, C. A comparison of flooding and thought stopping in the treatment of obsessional neurosis. *Behaviour Research and Therapy*, 1975, *13*, 263-269.

Hodgson, R. J., & Rachman, S. The effects of contamination and washing in obsessional patients. *Behaviour Research and Therapy*, 1972, *10*, 111-117.

Hodgson, R. J., & Rachman, S. Obsessional-compulsive complaints. *Behaviour Research and Therapy*, 1977, *15*, 389-395.

Ingram, I. M. Obsessional illness in mental hospital patients. *Journal of Mental Science*, 1961, *107*, 382-402.(a)

Ingram, I. M. Obsessional personality and anal-erotic character. *Journal of Mental Science*, 1961, *107*, 1035-1042.(b)

Insel, T. R., Gillin, J. C., Moore, A., Mendelson, W. B., Loewenstein, R. J., & Murphy, D. L. The sleep of patients with obsessive-compulsive disorder. *Archives of General Psychiatry*, 1982, *39*, 1372-1377.

Insel, T, Kalin, N. H., Guttmacher, L. B., Cohen, R. M., & Murphy, D. L. The Dexamethasone Suppression Test in patients with primary obsessive-compulsive disorder. *Psychiatry Research*, 1982, *6*, 153-160.

Kelly, D. *Anxiety and emotions: Physiological basis and treatment*. Springield, IL: Charles C Thomas, 1980.

Kirk, J. W. Behavioral treatment of obsessional-compulsive patients in routine clinical practice. *Behaviour Research and Therapy*, 1983, *21*, 57–62.

Kringlen, E. Obsessional neurotics: A long term follow-up. *British Journal of Psychiatry*, 1965, *111*, 709–722.

Lader, M. The peripheral and central role of the catecholamines in the mechanisms of anxiety. *Internal Journal of Pharmacopsychiatric Medicine*, 1974, *9*, 125–137.

Lader, M. H. Physiological research in anxiety. In H. M. van Praag (Ed.), *Research in neurosis*. New York: SP Medical & Scientific Books, 1978.

Lewis, A. J. Problems of obsessional illness. *Proceedings of the Royal Society of Medicine*, 1936, *29*, 325–336.

Lewis, A. J. Obsessional illness. *Acta Neuropsiquiátrica Argentina*, 1957, *3*, 323–335.

Lewis, A. J. Obsessional disorder. In R. Scott (Ed.), *Price's textbook of the practice of medicine* (10th ed.). London: Oxford University Press, 1966.

Lo, W. H. A follow-up study of obsessional neurotics in Hong Kong Chinese. *British Journal of Psychiatry*, 1967, *113*, 823–832.

Makhlouf-Norris, F., & Norris, H. The obsessive compulsive syndrome as a neurotic device for the reduction of self-uncertainty. *British Journal of Psychiatry*, 1972, *121*, 277–288.

Marks, I. M., Crowe, M., Drewe, E., Young, J., & Dewhurst, W. G. Obsessive compulsive neurosis in identical twins. *British Journal of Psychiatry*, 1969, *115*, 991–998.

Marks, I. M., Stern, R. S., Mawson, D., Cobb, J., & McDonald, R. Clomipramine and exposure for obsessive-compulsive rituals: I. *British Journal of Psychiatry*, 1980, *136*, 1–25, 1980.

Mavissakalian, M. Functional classification of obsessive-compulsive phenomena. *Journal of Behavioral Assessment*, 1979, *1*, 271–279.

Mavissakalian, M. Antidepressants in the treatment of agoraphobia and obsessive-compulsive disorder. *Comprehensive Psychiatry*, 1983, *24*(3), 278–284.

Mavissakalian, M. R., & Barlow, D. H. Assessment of obsessive-compulsive disorders. In D. H. Barlow (Ed.), *Behavioral assessment of adult disorders*. New York: Guilford Press, 1981.

Mavissakalian, M., & Michelson, L. Tricyclic antidepressants in obsessive-compulsive disorder: Antiobsessional or antidepressant agents? *Journal of Nervous and Mental Disease*, 1983, *171*, 301–306.

Mawson, D., Marks, I. M., & Ramm, L. Clomipramine and exposure for chronic obsessive-compulsive rituals: III. Two year follow-up and further findings. *British Journal of Psychiatry*, 1982, *140*, 11–18.

Monroe, S. M. Assessment of life events: Retrospective vs. concurrent strategies. *Archives of General Psychiatry*, 1982, *39*, 606–610.(a)

Monroe, S. M. Life events and disorder: Event-symptoms associations and the course of disorder. *Journal of Abnormal Psychology*, 1982, *91*, 14–24.(b)

Pollak, J. M. Obsessive-compulsive personality: A review. *Psychological Bulletin*, 1979, *86*, 225–241.

Rabavilas, A. D., & Boulougouris, J. C. Physiological accompaniments of ruminations, flooding, and thought stopping in obsessive patients. *Behaviour Research and Therapy*, 1974, *12*, 239–243.

Rabavilas, A. D., Boulougouris, J. C., Perissaka, C., & Stefanis, C. The effect of peripheral beta blockade on psychophysiologic responses in obsessional neurotics. *Comprehensive Psychiatry*, 1979, *20*, 378–383.

Rachman, S. Primary obsessional slowness. *Behaviour Research and Therapy*, 1974, *12*, 9–18.

Rachman, S. The modification of obsessions: A new formulation. *Behaviour Research and Therapy*, 1976, *14*, 437–443.

Rachman, S. The conditioning theory of fear acquisition: A critical examination. *Behaviour Research and Therapy*, 1977, *15*, 375–387.

Rachman, S., & de Silva, P. Abnormal and normal obsessions. *Behaviour Research and Therapy*, 1978, *16*, 233–248.

Rachman, S. J., & Hodgson, R. J. *Obsessions and compulsions*. Englewood Cliffs, NJ: Prentice-Hall, 1980.

Rachman, S., & Seligman, M. E. P. Unprepared phobias: "Be prepared." *Behaviour Research and Therapy*, 1976, *14*, 333–338.

Rachman, S., de Silva, P., & Roper, G. The spontaneous decay of compulsive urges. *Behaviour Research and Therapy*, 1976, *14*, 445–453.

Rachman, S., Cobb, J., Grey, S., MacDonald, B., Mawson, D., Sartory, G., & Stern, R. The behavioral treatment of obsessive-compulsive disorders, with or without clomipramine. *Behaviour Research and Therapy*, 1979, *17*, 467–468.

Reed, G. F. Some formal qualities of obsessional thinking. *Psychiatric Clinic*, 1968, *1*, 382–392.

Roper, G., & Rachman, S. Obsessional-compulsive checking: Experimental replication and development. *Behaviour Research and Therapy*, 1976, *14*, 25–32.

Roper, G., Rachman, S., & Hodgson, R. An experiment on obsessional checking. *Behaviour Research and Therapy*, 1973, *11*, 271–277.

Sartorius, N. Epidemiology of anxiety. *Pharmacopsychiatry*, 1980, *13*, 249–253.

Seligman, M. E. P. On generality of the laws of learning. *Psychological Review*, 1970, *77*, 406–418.

Seligman, M. E. P. Phobias and preparedness. *Behavior Therapy*, 1971, *2*, 307–320.

Seligman, M. E. P., & Hager, J. L. *Biological boundaries of learning*. Englewood Cliffs, NJ: Prentice-Hall, 1972.

Shields, J. *Genetic factors in neurosis.* In H. M. van Praag (Ed.), *Research in neurosis.* New York: SP Medical & Scientific Books, 1978.

Stern, R. S. Obsessive thought: The problem of therapy. *British Journal of Psychiatry,* 1978, *132,* 200–205.

Stern, R. S., & Cobb, J. P. Phenomenology of obsessive-compulsive neurosis. *British Journal of Psychiatry,* 1978, *132,* 233–239.

Stern, R. S., Lipsedge, M. S., & Marks, I. M. Obsessive ruminations: A controlled trial of thought-stopping technique. *Behaviour Research and Therapy,* 1973, *11,* 659–662.

Stern, R. S., Marks, I. M., Mawson, D., & Luscombe, D. K. Clomipramine and exposure for compulsive rituals: II. Plasma levels, side effects, and outcome. *British Journal of Psychiatry,* 1980, *136,* 161–166.

Thoren, P., Asberg, M., Cronholm, B., Jornestedt, L., & Traskman, L. Clomipramine treatment of obsessive-compulsive disorder. *Archives of General Psychiatry,* 1980, *37,* 1281–1285.(a)

Thoren, P., Asberg, M., Bertilsson, L., Mellstom, B., Sjoqvista, F., & Traskman, L. Clomipramine treatment of obsessive-compulsive disorder. *Archives of General Psychiatry,* 1980, *37,* 1289–1294.(b)

Turner, S. M. & Beidel, D. C. *Biological factors in obsessive-compulsive disorder.* University of Pittsburgh, unpublished manuscript, 1984.

Turner, S. M., Hersen, M., Bellack, A. S., Andrasik, F., & Capparell, H. V. Behavioral treatment of obsessive-compulsive neurosis. *Behaviour Research and Therapy,* 1979, *17,* 95–106.

Turner, S. M., Hersen, M., Bellack, A. S., Andrasik, F., & Capparell, H. V. Behavioral and pharmacological treatment of obsessive-compulsive disorders. *Journal of Nervous and Mental Disease,* 1980, *158,* 651–657.

Turner, S. M., Jacob, R. G., Beidel, D. C., & Himmelhoch, J. *Fluoxetine treatment of obsessive-compulsive disorder.* University of Pittsburgh, unpublished manuscript, 1984.

Walker, V. J., & Beech, H. R. Mood state and the ritualistic behavior of obsessional patients. *British Journal of Psychiatry,* 1969, *115,* 1261–1268.

Walton, D., & Mather, M. D. The application of learning principles to the treatment of obsessive-compulsive states in the acute and chronic phases of illness. *Behaviour Research and Therapy,* 1963, *2,* 163–174.

Wolpe, J. *Psychotherapy by reciprocal inhibition.* Stanford: Stanford University Press, 1958.

Index

249